W9-CIR-917

Talking with Patients and Families about Medical Error

Talking with Patients and Families about Medical Error

A Guide for Education and Practice

ROBERT D. TRUOG, M.D.
DAVID M. BROWNING, M.S.W., B.C.D., F.T.
JUDITH A. JOHNSON, J.D.
THOMAS H. GALLAGHER, M.D.

Foreword by Lucian L. Leape, M.D.

Prepared in Cooperation
with The Risk Management Foundation
of the Harvard Medical Institutions, Inc.

The Johns Hopkins University Press

Baltimore

Research and practical application of the guidelines outlined in *Talking with Patients and Families about Medical Error* was funded primarily by CRICO, the medical malpractice insurer for the Harvard Medical Institutions.

Printed in the United States of America on acid-free paper
9 8 7 6 5 4 3 2 1

The Johns Hopkins University Press
2715 North Charles Street
Baltimore, Maryland 21218-4363
www.press.jhu.edu

Library of Congress Cataloging-in-Publication Data

Talking with patients and families about medical error : a guide for education and practice / Robert D. Truog . . . [et al.]; foreword by Lucian L. Leape.
p. ; cm.
Includes bibliographical references and index.
ISBN-13: 978-0-8018-9804-4 (hardcover : alk. paper)
ISBN-10: 0-8018-9804-8 (hardcover : alk. paper)
1. Medical errors. 2. Physician and patient. 3. Communication in medicine. I. Truog, Robert.
[DNLM: 1. Physician-Patient Relations. 2. Medical Errors. 3. Truth Disclosure. W 62 T1465 2011]
R729.8.T35 2011
610—dc22 2010013268

A catalog record for this book is available from the British Library.

Special discounts are available for bulk purchases of this book. For more information, please contact Special Sales at 410-516-6936 or specialsales@press.jhu.edu.

The Johns Hopkins University Press uses environmentally friendly book materials, including recycled text paper that is composed of at least 30 percent post-consumer waste, whenever possible. All of our book papers are acid-free, and our jackets and covers are printed on paper with recycled content.

Contents

Foreword, by Lucian L. Leape, M.D. vii
Acknowledgments xi
Introduction xiii

1 Medical Error through the Eyes of Clinicians, Patients, and Families 1
2 What Is a Medical Error? 10
3 A Brief Overview of the Patient Safety Movement 16
4 Communicating about Adverse Events and Medical Error 31
5 Supporting Clinicians in Disclosure: *The Coaching Model* 57
6 Practice-Based Learning for Coaches and Clinicians 64
7 Practical Guidelines for Disclosure 74
8 Learning through Enacting 92
9 The Broad Spectrum of Adverse Events and Medical Error 103
10 Organizational Strategies for Improving Disclosure Practice 118
11 Future Directions and Closing Thoughts 131

Appendix: *Practical Guidelines for Disclosure* 139
Annotated Bibliography of Key Works 141
References 155
Index 167

Foreword

Lucian L. Leape, M.D.

The driving concept behind the modern patient safety movement is simple and powerful: errors are caused by bad systems, not by bad people. Actualizing this notion has proceeded in two major directions: creating a non-punitive environment where it is safe to report and talk about mistakes and making changes to the bad systems. Success in both dimensions has been highly variable, and at times slow, although there have been some spectacular successes, such as the virtual elimination of certain types of hospital-acquired infections.

Coincident with the increase in awareness of the extent of preventable medical injury, and undoubtedly facilitated by the discussion of efforts to change systems, has been the rise of patient advocacy groups, such as Consumers Advancing Patient Safety (CAPS), Medically Induced Trauma Support Services (MITSS), Persons United Limiting Substandards and Errors in Health Care (PULSE), the Josie King Foundation, and Mothers Against Medical Errors (MAME).These organizations have been founded by individuals who were injured by or who lost a loved one to a medical error. Although most of these organizations seek to improve the safety of medical care, the stories the founders tell are less about injury and mistakes and more about how they were treated when things went wrong. The common themes are stonewalling of information, refusal to take responsibility, and refusal to admit error or apologize. Thus, the major focus for these groups has been on efforts to improve communication and support. Rather than sue, they seek to mobilize public opinion to force change.

The time is ripe for change. We have long known that a serious medical mishap is devastating for the patient, imposing an immense emotional burden on top of the physical suffering and fracturing the trust that is the cornerstone of the doctor-patient relationship. And we know that honesty, transparency, and apology are essential to ease that burden and rebuild that trust. Yet, too often it doesn't happen. In no aspect of health care is the discrepancy between what is known and what is practiced greater than it is in communicating with patients when things go wrong. Most doctors, I believe, are honest and communicate well with their patients. But too many do not, as the horrendous annual number of malpractice suits bears witness. Why?

The reasons are complex, as you will come to understand reading this book. For decades, doctors and hospitals have been given bad advice by their lawyers, who have been more concerned (incorrectly, it turns out) about our liability than our humanity. But this advice to deny responsibility and avoid apology was not totally unwelcome to physicians. It fed into their fears of shame and disgrace and provided cover for avoiding the painful discussion with the patient and the revelation of fallibility. A complex psychology, abetted by longstanding peer-sanctioned tradition.

Sadly, disclosure malfunction is but one example of a much larger problem: the dysfunctional culture of most health care institutions. For every instance of a patient who is lied to—for that is what failing to admit to and explain a serious medical error is—there are multiple instances of disrespectful treatment as well as disruptive, disrespectful, and even abusive conduct toward nurses, residents, and medical students. And even more instances of subtle, insidious, even institutionalized disrespect. Again, this is not the majority of physicians—far from it—but it is enough to "poison the well" and create an atmosphere of fear and distrust. No wonder that creating a non-punitive environment where doctors and nurses can safely report and discuss their errors has proved so difficult to achieve or that working together in interdisciplinary teams has also proved difficult. Changing that culture has been the daunting challenge of the safety movement.

In this context, the insights and recommendations by Robert Truog, David Browning, Judith Johnson, and Thomas Gallagher provide guidance not only for improving communication with patients at their time of special need but also for the deeper and more pervasive cultural changes that our sick systems so sorely need. For example, we have learned that improving patient safety is less about implementing new practices than about building the relationships that make implementation possible. Relationships, the authors wisely remind us, are guided and formed by our values. The core values they identify as essential to rebuilding relationships after a mishap—transparency, respect, accountability, continuity, and kindness—are in fact the core values needed to build relationships in the first place, not just between providers and patients but among all caregivers and workers in our hospitals. Making these values explicit and working to incorporate them in response to a serious event can be, and I predict will be, a powerful "entering wedge" for making the deeper cultural changes our institutions need.

So, if all it does is to help the reader begin to change the conversation about the culture of our medical institutions, this book will make a substantial contribution. Fortunately for those seeking help in dealing with disclosure, it provides much more. In addition to addressing the specifics of communicating with and supporting patients and caregivers after an event—the 34 guidelines alone make it a treasure—the authors center their advice in the context of the needs of the patients and their caregivers. The discussion of coaching and the many scenarios of error disclosure provide a wealth of examples of the types of challenges that must be confronted in learning the complex skills of communicating when things go wrong.

But this is much more than a "how to" manual. Early on, the authors emphasize that communication between caregiver and patient is more about feelings than words, more about heart than methods. The truth of this concept is manifest in the context and tone of what you are about to read, enhancing and giving power to the wise words of advice that follow.

Acknowledgments

In offering this guide to talking with patients and families about medical error, the authors would like to acknowledge and thank all of those patients, families, and professionals who have contributed to the effort to promote transparency, accountability, and fairness in the response of clinicians and institutions to unanticipated events and medical errors. In addition, we thank our colleagues at the Institute for Professionalism and Ethical Practice, and in particular Drs. Elaine Meyer, Elizabeth Rider, and Sigall Bell, for their insights and support of the educational approach and methods embraced by this book.

All of the authors received grant support from CRICO/RMF. In addition, Dr. Gallagher's work was supported by the Agency for Healthcare Research and Quality (1RO1HS016506, 1U18HS016658), the Robert Wood Johnson Foundation Investigator Award in Health Policy Research program, and the Greenwall Foundation. Ms. Johnson's work was also supported by Harvard Medical School.

This book would not have been possible without the support of CRICO/RMF. Since 1976, CRICO/RMF has served the Harvard medical community by providing malpractice insurance as well as tools to promote patient safety and quality improvement. RMF Strategies was created to reach beyond the borders of the Harvard community to create new partnerships among physicians, healthcare systems, and their medical malpractice insurers, using what works: comparing analysis of claims data, sharing effective patient safety practice, and promoting dialogue among a national community of peers. Most recently, it has focused on the development of multifaceted tools, including this book, to assist healthcare systems in developing effective programs that support clinicians in disclosure and apology after adverse events and medical errors. For more information, visit www.rmf.harvard.edu and www.rmfstrategies.com.

Introduction

Over the past decade or so, issues of patient safety and the prevention of medical error have become one of the most important topics in the practice of medicine. The shocking discovery that medical error is one of the leading causes of death in the United States has galvanized the medical profession, the public, and third-party payers into a unprecedented coalition for patient safety advocacy.[1]

Fundamental to the patient safety movement has been the insight that the current culture of medicine not only fails to promote quality improvement and safety but effectively impedes its development and progress. The strong historical emphasis on personal responsibility has fostered the view that patient safety depends on ferreting out and eliminating the "bad apples," those who lack either the personal character or the knowledge to provide good medical care. This bad apple mentality has helped to create a culture of silence in health care regarding errors in which health care workers hesitate to report errors to their health care organization or discuss them with colleagues lest they be seen as the bad apple that needs to be removed from the barrel. Health care workers' silence regarding errors has made it difficult to learn about the true causes of medical errors or to develop effective prevention strategies.

This bad apple view is gradually being supplanted by the more nuanced concept that medical errors occur within a complex, interdependent system of medical care. There is broad consensus that the most effective way to make health care safer is not to identify and punish the failure of individuals (although in some egregious cases, such action will still be necessary) but to encourage the broad sharing of information and knowledge about adverse events that can then lead to systems changes. In addition to advocating for greater openness within the profession itself, more progressive thinkers have encouraged clinicians and institutions to reach out to patients and families as well, partnering with them through the sharing of information and involving them in the overall mission of enhancing patient safety.

The many threads that have been woven into the patient safety movement will be explored in greater detail below, but no matter how effective this effort becomes, medicine will never be perfect, and adverse events and medical errors will always be a part of health care. Furthermore, studies now reveal that the pain and suffering experienced by those who are involved in these events come not just from the medical consequences themselves but from the way that these events are disclosed and discussed. In particular, we are discovering that the conversations that occur between patients, families, and clinicians in the aftermath of an adverse event or error can have a profound impact on everyone involved.

This observation was emphasized in an article coauthored by Hillary Clinton and Barack Obama in the *New England Journal of Medicine* in 2006. In the context of malpractice reform, they noted: "Studies show that the most important factor in people's decisions to file lawsuits is not negligence, but ineffective communication between patients and providers."[2] While this point may seem relatively obvious and unsurprising, on close examination it reveals an insight that is critical for the patient safety movement. Lawsuits are not driven simply by the occurrence of medical error. Most errors, even serious errors, are never litigated. A common precipitant of lawsuits following medical errors is the perception of patients and families that they were not treated well, that clinicians failed to communicate effectively or compassionately with them, and that the clinicians failed to learn any lessons that might prevent the error from happening to others in the future.

Often, existing relationships between clinicians and patients are ruptured at the time of an error, never to be repaired. While lawsuits are sometimes the inevitable pathway to the legal resolution of these events, they rarely adequately address the psychological pain and suffering experienced by the patients, families, and clinicians involved. The purpose of this book is to explore the critical yet exceptionally difficult conversations that follow adverse events and error, in the knowledge that these conversations can play an important role in whether those who are involved experience healing and closure or carry anger and guilt for the rest of their lives.

As with any difficult conversation, whether between a physician and patient or between friends or family members, simple rules have only limited utility. Health care workers endorse the principle of being open with patients following errors but are unsure how to turn this principle into practice. Advice such as "tell the truth" or "be compassionate" may be helpful but is usually inadequate. Commonly the "truth" of an event is open to a wide range of interpretation, and memorized phrases designed to communicate compassion often sound wooden and can make matters even worse. Furthermore, while the content of the conversation is important, *how* something is said can have as much impact as precisely *what* is said.

This book represents a synthesis of what we have learned from the research that has been performed on this topic as well as the knowledge we have gained through the development of numerous educational presentations, workshops, and lectures that the authors have created with colleagues at Harvard Medical School, the University of Washington, and Washington University in St. Louis. This material has been taught in a variety of venues and formats, including workshops involving more than 400 participants at Harvard Medical School under the auspices of the Harvard Risk Management Foundation, as well as several hundred presentations to other audiences both nationally and internationally. Our goal is to provide a comprehensive method, encompassing both organizational strategies and individual advice, to improve the performance of clinicians in communicating with patients and families in the aftermath of an adverse event or medical error.

Instead of approaching this topic through abstract conceptual or theoretical considerations, we frame our treatment of this subject in terms of the lived experiences of those who are involved in the process—the patients, their families, doctors, nurses, social workers, chaplains, and others. We therefore begin our discussion in Chapter 1 by looking at medical error through the eyes of clinicians, patients, and families. Here we recount several narratives that explore the experience of medical error from a variety of perspectives.

In Chapter 2 we explore a variety of approaches that have been taken toward defining medical error and discuss the terminology we use in this book. In the next chapter we provide a brief overview of the patient safety movement, which sets the stage for the material that follows by framing the topic of disclosure within the broader context of quality and patient safety. We describe the ways that government, academia, the health care industry, and advocacy groups have shaped the history of this movement and how these developments impact our approach to these difficult conversations.

In Chapter 4, we narrow our focus to the topic of communicating about adverse events and medical error. Here we closely examine the tradition of nondisclosure within health care, the development of ethical and professional norms that are slowly changing this tradition, and the research that has examined the needs and desires of patients, families, and clinicians who are involved in medical errors. Finally, we explore the creation and evolution of programs and policies designed to support clinicians in the process of disclosing these events to patients and families.

Chapter 5 is focused on the "coaching model," the paradigm we have chosen to structure the context of disclosure conversations. This model, which has been endorsed by the National Quality Forum, is predicated on the observation that literally hundreds of individuals within each institution need to be skilled in having difficult conversations about medical errors when these unfortunate circumstances arise. On the assumption that it is not practical or feasible to keep all of them knowledgeable and trained all of the time, we suggest that organizations rely on a cohort of coaches who can provide "just-in-time" guidance and advice to their fellow clinicians on a 24/7 basis.

This book therefore addresses disclosure at two levels. First, we cover the nuts-and-bolts advice that any clinician needs to be able to have skillful conversations with patients and families. Second, we discuss the unique skills that coaches must have in order to be able to provide the solid support necessary for other clinicians to have these conversations. Although these roles overlap to a large extent, certain aspects are distinct, and the book is structured to cover both.

Chapter 6, "Practice-based Learning for Coaches and Clinicians," describes a methodology for teaching clinicians these new communication practices. First, we define the core relational values that inform these skills—values that build (and rebuild) health care relationships. Second, we discuss the importance of providing a compassionate and empathic response to others that is sensitive to the emotional impact of these events. Third, we explore the role and importance of apology. Fourth, we examine how to approach these conversations as collaborative and interactive events. Fifth, we explain the importance of perspective taking—that is, seeing these events through the lenses of the patients, families, clinicians, and the organizational culture that surrounds them.

With this as background, in Chapter 7 we provide concrete advice, presented as bullet points, for individuals who are about to have these conversations and for the coaches who are supporting them. We specifically address issues such as the first priorities that need attention after an adverse event and how to prepare for the initial conversation with the patient and family, and we provide recommendations for the conversation itself, along with advice regarding documentation and follow-up.

In the next chapter, "Learning through Enacting," we present our experience with teaching disclosure skills by means of a hypothetical case of a medication error that led to a respiratory arrest. In this scenario, the error is quickly recognized and addressed, and the patient makes a full recovery. When using this exercise, we ask several participants to play the roles of those involved in the event and to engage in a conversation about this error with professional actors who are in the roles of the patient and her husband. We have found this exercise to be very effective at enabling clinicians to translate their commitment to transparency into action.

A fascinating (and unanticipated) finding from these enactments has been the widely divergent approaches taken by the participants from one workshop to another. This process has given us insight into the variety of styles, assumptions, and principles that guide different clinicians in facing these challenging conversations. These insights have led us to understand an important pedagogical principle that has become a strong philosophical foundation of our educational approach, namely, that the ability to communicate empathy, compassion, and concern cannot be learned through the acquisition of communication "skills"—understood as techniques such as the use of body language and carefully selected words and phrases in the practice of conversation. The teaching of these skills has become quite popular within the customer service industries, where they may be sufficient to give the appearance of genuine caring and engagement, even in the absence of any true relational connection. In our view, while these approaches may be effective for providers in fast-food restaurants or on telephone help lines, they often fail miserably in the context of the patient-clinician relationship, where patients and families quickly realize when they are being handled or managed. Our focus is therefore on the values and attitudes that underlie these conversations. In particular, we emphasize five features of the relationship that deserve special attention: transparency, respect, accountability, continuity, and kindness (constituting the acronym TRACK), features that articulate these values and have served as a useful foundation for the heart of our teaching.

Despite the usefulness of concrete advice, however, no two situations are ever the same, and the ability to conduct these conversations skillfully will always remain something of an art form, with some individuals more innately talented than others. Furthermore, no rules or principles can ever completely capture all of the nuance and subtlety surrounding issues such as when it might be ethically acceptable to withhold information from patients and families, the correct amount of detail to be communicated in any situation, or the best approaches for responding to anger, denial, or sarcasm. In Chapter 9 we present a spectrum of hypothetical cases, ranging from the trivial to the tragic, from inpatient to outpatient settings, and across a variety of disciplines, and use these cases to discuss some of the many facets of how such cases may be approached and successfully addressed.

Up to this point, a fair criticism of the book could be that many of the recommendations we suggest cannot be implemented without transformational organizational change. We address this in Chapter 10 by taking a close look at organizational strategies that are effective—indeed necessary—for improving disclosure practice. We structure this discussion within the "4-A Framework for Organizational Disclosure Strategies," focusing on awareness, accountability, ability, and action.

Our final chapter looks to the future and envisions some of the developments that we anticipate in the years to come. These include efforts to link disclosure quality and safety programs, better understanding of and support for the needs of patients and clinicians alike, and innovative approaches to early compensation for some types of medical injury as well as strategies to address the common situation when the hospital and the physician staff do not share the same malpractice carrier. We make recommendations for changes to the reporting structure of the National Practitioner Data Bank that would enhance disclosure, and we look for the development of ever more creative and effective methods for improving the ability of clinicians to engage in these challenging conversations.

Finally, given the burgeoning literature on this topic, we have appended an annotated bibliography to serve as a reference and a guide to some of the more important and influential works that exist, in print and online, in this relatively new but already complex area of medical practice.

Talking with Patients and Families about Medical Error

ONE

Medical Error through the Eyes of Clinicians, Patients, and Families

We begin with a story that illustrates dramatically the impact of medical error on patients and families. It involves a professional violinist who had been diagnosed with colon cancer. The following dialogue is taken from separate interviews with the patient, prior to his death, and with his wife and adult son. They describe a cascading series of disappointments that include faulty communication, complications from procedures, adverse events, and medical errors. In his first hospitalization, the patient underwent a partial colectomy, which was complicated by perforation of the ileum. He was discharged with undiagnosed pneumonia and then rehospitalized, at which time he fell while being transferred between hospital units. He was later hospitalized again to remove the colostomy. The procedure was unsuccessful, and he died four days later. The following are excerpts of the story as told by the patient, his wife, and son:

PATIENT

I think the head surgeon was lost. He approached me—I don't want to say this badly—as if I were a piece of meat that he had just sewn up. If I would ask him a direct question, I would get, we might say, an indirect answer. For example my colostomy, I asked him, would I have to live with it or could I have another operation, and his answer would be, that's up to me [the patient]. Well, I mean, I don't know enough to make such a decision . . . In terms of compassion or understanding another person's sensitivity, he did not make any effort to do that with me.

You have no idea how far a "sorry" will go . . . As to what I'm going to do about it, I don't think there's anything I can do. There is no recourse. I'm not aware that I, in the role of a patient, have any power at all.

WIFE

No one ever said they were sorry. You know, that's what happens in medicine. They didn't say that, they just never attended to that. No one ever apologized for the condition he was in. Not at all. I wouldn't mind suing the hospital.

SON

The complications that occurred were of such enormity that it really took the wind from all of our lungs. It was almost as if a tornado came in and out, and by the time the tornado left, there was a whole wake of questions, and conflicts, and emotional traumas and dramas.

If anybody would have acknowledged some accountability, an apology, to actually reach out and connect with us on human terms—in human language. Not legalese, not the legality of a letter, primarily a sense that they were sorry, and that there is a willingness for them to be vulnerable enough to acknowledge that there might be an imperfection in the system. And, to acknowledge, by accountability, that the system can change.

My mother wrote a letter to the hospital, and in that letter she discussed her concerns regarding my father's care. All she got back was a phone call asking if she planned to pursue a lawsuit. My mother became furious when she received copies of bills indicating that our insurance companies have paid the hospital hundreds and hundreds of thousands of dollars for the care we felt led to our father's death.

The objective of a lawsuit is never, for me, about a monetary gain. It is for the education of the system. It is to put the system under a microscope such that the system itself can benefit . . .

Time heals, but it doesn't heal when there are so many questions that have not been answered. And that's a very difficult thing for us still to be dealing with.

This narrative captures the diverse ways in which trust and communication can break down between patients, families, and clinicians. It reveals the absence of transparency and respect coming from clinicians, the lack of accountability and continuity on the part of the hospital, and the dearth of kindness shown throughout the process. The case characteristically includes multiple missed opportunities over many months when clinicians and other hospital delegates might have initiated some repair to the damaged relationship with the patient and family, opportunities that appear to have been botched or simply not pursued.

Patients and families are not the only ones impacted by medical error, however. One of the pioneers in promoting greater transparency regarding medical error was Dr. David Hilfiker, a family physician who practiced in a small town in Minnesota. In 1984, he submitted some personal reflections about one of his cases for possible publication in the *New England Journal of Medicine.*[3] In his narrative, he described a horrific medical error in which he performed a D&C abortion on a woman for what he mistakenly believed to be a case of fetal demise with failed miscarriage but what in fact turned out to be an otherwise healthy fetus. In a show of remarkable candor for that era, he openly shared the truth of what happened with the woman and her husband. While he fully acknowledged in the essay the profound suffering he had caused this family, his purpose in writing the narrative was to describe the pain of the event from the perspective of a physician and to generalize from his experience to the ways that both medical culture and society have traditionally viewed these acts of personal failure on the part of clinicians. A few of his observations follow:

> The potential consequences of our medical mistakes are so overwhelming that it is almost impossible for practicing physicians to deal with their errors in a psychologically healthy fashion. Most people—doctors and patients alike—harbor deep within themselves the expectation that the physician will be perfect. No one seems prepared to accept the simple fact of life that physicians, like anyone else, will make mistakes.
>
> The drastic consequences of our mistakes, the repeated opportunities to make them, the uncertainty about our own culpability when

results are poor, and the medical and societal denial that mistakes must happen all result in an intolerable paradox for the physician. We see the horror of our own mistakes, yet we are given no permission to deal with their enormous emotional impact; instead, we are forced to continue the routine of repeatedly making decisions, any one of which could lead us back into the same pit.

At some point we must bring our mistakes out of the closet. We need to give ourselves permission to recognize our errors and their consequences. We need to find healthy ways to deal with our emotional responses to those errors. Our profession is difficult enough without having to wear the yoke of perfection.

Initially the editors of the *New England Journal of Medicine* attempted to dissuade Hilfiker from publishing the piece, advising him of the irreparable damage that such a story could cause for him, personally and professionally. He courageously pushed forward with sharing his story, and the narrative has become a classic, both for its message and for the influence it has had on initiating a shift in the cultural attitudes within medicine that had made the subject of medical error taboo for centuries.[4]

For many physicians and nurses, their own experiences with medical error have had a significant and lasting influence on their personal and professional development. One of the authors (Robert Truog) was involved in one such event more than twenty years ago during his residency training in pediatrics. This is the story he tells as a part of the workshops that we have conducted:

One evening, when I was working as a junior pediatrics resident, I saw a 9-month-old boy who had cold symptoms and a temperature of 104. I drew blood for a culture and a complete blood count and gave him some Tylenol. I went to see some other patients and checked in on him about thirty minutes later. By that point, his fever was down and he was playful and interactive, so I sent him home with a diagnosis of a viral upper respiratory infection.

The next morning, the lab called to say that the boy's blood culture was growing gram-positive diplococci. His parents brought him back in, and we admitted him to the intensive care unit with what we ultimately learned was pneumococcal sepsis and meningitis.

He survived but was neurologically devastated. Ultimately, we discharged him to a rehabilitation hospital with a tracheostomy and a feeding tube.

That same morning, the chief resident called me to her office and asked, "Bob, what happened here?" I explained my actions, confused as to why my judgment was being called into question. Then she pressed me, "Yes, but what about his white blood cell count?" It was at that moment that I realized I had drawn blood for a CBC but had forgotten to check the results. In fact, the white count was over 40,000 with a left shift; if I had looked at that result, I would never have sent this little boy home, let alone neglected to give him antibiotics.

I was devastated, and surprised by what happened next. The chief resident looked sympathetically at me and said, "Bob, you've been a good resident—this isn't typical for you. It would be a bad thing if this got out among your colleagues in the program and the faculty. So why don't we plan to keep this between you and me . . . and never let it happen again." I felt very grateful and agreed with her assessment—it would be terrible for me professionally if this error for which I was responsible came out in the open.

I went on to become chief resident myself, and I admitted that little boy several times over the next few years when he would develop aspiration pneumonias. My friends and colleagues never knew the story behind the story, and the family, of course, never learned what had happened. When I left the hospital and moved to another part of the country, I lost track of him. But I've wondered many times over the past twenty years whether he is still alive and about how my error impacted him and his family.

Although no one today would attempt to argue that this case was handled well, it does provide an opportunity to reflect on what has changed and what is still pretty much the same. Much has improved; systems have been put into place to minimize the chance of important laboratory results being overlooked, and junior trainees are more consistently supervised by attending physicians. More broadly there is an increasingly open atmosphere in health care organizations about mistakes, a growing shift toward recognizing the role that system breakdowns play in most medical errors, and a greater willingness on the part of health care organizations to examine mistakes that occur.

Yet other aspects of the problem seem to have changed very little. Clinicians are still reluctant to go out of their way to disclose errors to patients and families who may be too intimidated or unsophisticated to ask the right questions. Most clinicians who are more than a decade beyond their training have been taught to be extremely cautious when communicating with patients about errors: do not explicitly admit to errors, and if patients or families persist in asking questions about what happened, politely refrain from providing detailed explanations and refer them to the office of legal counsel, if necessary. Indeed, hospitals have developed elaborate peer-protected review mechanisms to prevent patients and their attorneys from accessing certain types of information pertaining to the analysis of medical errors. Sometimes this withholding of information about errors has been framed as a benevolent act, much like not informing a patient of a terminal diagnosis due to concern that such information might cause the patient to give up hope.

This narrative also illustrates another tension that emerges in these situations—the role of professional collegiality, friendship, and loyalty within health care. Involvement in medical error can have a devastating effect on professional careers. Almost everyone who has spent a significant amount of time in health care has seen someone who suffered significant professional setbacks from his or her role in an error, sometimes far out of proportion to the actual degree of his or her culpability in the event. In addition to this professional impact, clinicians who are involved may suffer disabling psychological trauma, sometimes requiring prolonged periods of rehabilitation, which in extreme cases may preclude them from ever being able to return to their clinical roles.

Given that health care aspires to be a caring profession, what roles should friendship and loyalty play in the way that these events are handled? In the narrative related above, the chief resident almost certainly did protect the young resident from what likely would have been harsh consequences as a result of his error. But such loyalty and protection came at a steep price, in terms of the cost to the patient and his family, as well as the health care system in general, which missed an opportunity to learn from this instance of a missed lab result and the chance to potentially improve the system, thereby protecting future patients from the same tragic outcome.

Change has been slow, and even today the personal stories of clinicians continue to be a powerful force in shaping and driving the patient safety agenda. In 2008, Dr. David Rattner, chief of general and gastrointestinal surgery at Massachusetts General Hospital, volunteered to be interviewed on video about a medical error in which he was the protagonist:

> *It was a wrong site surgery case—a laterality issue, where the medical record had said one thing and the lesion was on the other. It was very bizarre because I'd always been afraid something like that could happen, but when it was happening, I just didn't have a clue that it was happening.*
>
> *When I took out the gland and I was told it was a normal gland, and went back and looked at the x-rays and looked at the report, I felt really foolish. I felt really terrible—it was not a happy moment.*
>
> *I decided, as part of this, that I would take greater interest in patient safety efforts . . . I volunteered to serve on several committees here having to do with patient safety . . . I made it an issue.*
>
> *That's the thing about this case I guess that's so incredible. Of all people for it to happen to, I would never have thought that I would have been the one. I was not the fastest. I was not the one racing through a huge schedule every day. I thought I had pretty good documentation. And then it happened. So, if it could happen to me, it certainly could happen to anybody.*

The preceding discussion of the impact of medical error on clinicians is not meant to imply that this is of more importance than the effect of such errors on patients and families, and it is certainly not an attempt to "blame the victim." These stories do highlight, however, the traditional reluctance to acknowledge the impact of medical error on clinicians. Indeed, with greater recognition of the fact that medical errors are often the result of systems failures, some commentators have suggested that the involved clinicians are sometimes quite literally the "second victims" of these events.[5] In any case, there is no doubt that our frequent failure to help clinicians to cope with these events on a personal level contributes to their failure to address these issues with their patients and to successfully maintain or restore the patient-clinician relationship.

As is detailed in Chapter 3, however, progress is being made. In 2006 the Harvard teaching hospitals collaborated on a consensus document entitled *When Things Go Wrong: Responding to Adverse Events*.[6] This landmark document courageously articulated a principle that many would regard as obvious but which few were previously willing to endorse—that communicating with patients and families is "the right thing to do." Beyond this important statement, however, the document provided few details about how to do this well. The final story, again from one of the authors (Robert Truog), shows how even good intentions are sometimes not good enough.

We had admitted to the ICU a 3-year-old child with leukemia who had developed typhlitis, an inflammation of the cecum, related to his immunosuppression. We had discussed his care in detail with the oncology team that had been caring for him on the ward. The following morning on rounds I was comparing his medication list with the recommendations from the oncologists and noted that whereas they had recommended 2 mg/kg of Solu-Medrol, we had written him for only 1 mg/kg. Although I knew this was medically insignificant under the circumstances, we made the change in his orders and went on.

That afternoon I stopped by his bed space to speak with his father. I updated him on all of his son's problems and reassured him that we were working closely with the oncologists. I made offhand mention of the fact that we had doubled the dose of steroids that we had given him the night before in response to the oncologists' recommendations. I was about to go on when he stopped me short.

"Wait!" he said. "You mean to tell me that he only got half as much steroids as he should have last night? The steroids are a critical part of his chemotherapy. I can't believe that you messed this up. How could this have happened? This is a famous Harvard hospital. What's going on here? Obviously, I can no longer trust you. My wife and I are going to have to be at his bedside 24 hours a day and

review every medication to make sure that you don't make another mistake."

I tried to explain to him that this event was absolutely inconsequential in terms of his son's care, even suggesting that that the error might have been a good thing, since he was already so immunosuppressed and a lower dose of steroids might help him in fighting an infection. Not surprisingly, he accused me of being defensive. By this time he was in constant motion, walking back and forth around the bed space, wringing his hands. At times he would slow down, and he would say things like, "I know you didn't need to tell me this, and I'm glad you were honest with me, but I still can't believe that something like this could have happened!"

The conversation did not have a good ending. After about 45 minutes I excused myself and told him that I would be back to talk more later. We had many more conversations, but without any resolution. Unfortunately, his son did not survive that admission, and I'm sure there will always be at least some question in his mind as to whether our error in steroid dosing may have played a role in that.

I left the room very confused. I truly believed that we should be honest with patients about medical errors. Yet this event made me realize that in these conversations honesty is just a piece of the puzzle.

Skillful, empathic conversations with patients and families require more than just openness and good intentions. While some cases may be destined to go poorly regardless of how they are handled, this case contained many opportunities for improvement, and the unskillful disclosure led to a breakdown in trust that was never repaired. The message of this case is really the purpose of this book. Conversations in the aftermath of adverse events and medical error are extremely difficult and complicated, yet knowledge of certain principles and guidelines can improve the capacity of clinicians to engage them with skill and confidence.

TWO

What Is a Medical Error?

This book is about difficult conversations that occur in the aftermath of adverse events and medical error. In order to properly frame the principles and guidance that we recommend, however, some background discussion of definitions, historical considerations, and conceptual distinctions is necessary.

Although the patient safety movement has matured considerably over the past several years, efforts to create a common set of definitions, categories, and concepts have not been uniformly successful. In fact, the image of the Tower of Babel has been invoked to illustrate that "a bewildering language of medical error and iatrogenic injury has evolved."[7]

In one of the seminal works on the nature of human error *(Human Error)*, James Reason offered the following working definition: "Error will be taken as a generic term to encompass all those occasions in which a planned sequence of mental or physical activities fails to achieve its intended outcome, and when these failures cannot be attributed to the intervention of some chance agency."[8] Reason goes on to describe ways of classifying errors, including the categories of "active" and "latent" errors. His work, particularly his understanding of the nature and complexity of latent (or systems) errors, has been very influential in health care.

Against this backdrop, several definitions of medical error have appeared in connection with patient safety. The Agency for Healthcare Research and Quality (AHRQ) considers medical error to include "an action taken" or "an action that is not taken" that results in or has the potential to result in harm to patients. The AHRQ further refers to common categories of errors such as "active failures" versus "latent conditions," and "slips" versus "mistakes." The federal Quality Interagency Coordination (QuIC) Task Force focuses on whether the event is preventable, treating medical errors as "adverse events that are preventable with our current state of medical knowledge." This idea is reflected in one of the most concise definitions of medical error, used by a number of leaders in the patient safety movement, as "a preventable adverse medical event."[9]

Other definitions focus on how to determine whether an error has occurred. For example, Smith and Forster propose that an action (or inaction) is a medical error if so characterized by "skilled and knowledgeable peers."[10] They further divide medical errors into one of three categories: errors of skill, rule, or knowledge. While they use the term to include only unintentional acts, they include in their definition mistakes that are "caught" before the patient is harmed.

In an article in *Nursing Ethics*, Nancy Crigger discusses a number of the more common definitions of medical error and then proposes four characteristics of medical error from an ethical point of view: (1) there is lack of intentionality (malevolent acts/omissions are not "mistakes"); (2) harm is not required (though such harm may be required to show legal negligence); (3) there is an element of "choice" (predetermined acts cannot involve "mistake"), and (4) there is responsibility (culpability), based on the element of choice.[11]

In addition to being aware of the different ways in which medical error is defined by scholars in the field, health-related government, and private organizations, it is important to note that individual clinicians and patients may have their own views on what constitutes an error. For example, in a study of operating room team members (nurses, anesthesiologists, surgeons) and patients, all respondents talked about error as a "deviation from standards of practice."[12] In this study, when the standard of care seemed ambiguous, participants were more apt to talk about an accident, "act of God," or "honest mistake." In these circumstances, they were also more apt to consider the seriousness of an adverse outcome in deciding whether an error had occurred.

Some studies have shown that patients may differ from clinicians in their views of what constitutes an error. For example, patients appear to have a broader concept of error, which includes breakdowns in the patient-provider relationship and difficulty in accessing care,[13] poor communication and interpersonal skills, and poor service generally.[14,15] In another study of patients' responses to self-identified "mistakes," patients interpreted a variety of actions as errors—including failure to pass on telephone messages, inability to get timely appointments, rudeness, and lack of time and attention.[16]

In contrast to "error," the term "adverse event" refers to any injury caused by medical management rather than by the patient's underlying disease. For example, the QuIC Task Force follows Leape and colleagues[17] in defining an adverse event as "an injury . . . caused by medical management [that] resulted in measurable disability."[9] The American Society for Healthcare Risk Management (ASHRM) uses the term "adverse event" to refer to a negative or bad result stemming from diagnostic, medical or surgical care. ASHRM also uses other terms, such as "unanticipated outcome" (and sometimes "unwelcome" outcome) to refer to an outcome of care significantly different from what was expected. None of these definitions presupposes that an adverse event is the result of error, is preventable, or implies legal liability. AHRQ is even more explicit on this point, noting that identifying an occurrence as an adverse event (that is, any injury caused by medical care) does not imply error or negligence.

Contributing to the confusion is the fact that "adverse event" and similar terms have very specific meanings under various state and federal laws (e.g., the meaning of adverse event under federal regulations requiring the reporting of certain unexpected medication problems in clinical research, the vaccine reporting laws, and various state laws requiring reporting of certain adverse events) and as used by health-related organizations (e.g., the Joint Commission, which has a specific definition of a reportable "sentinel event").

For our purposes in this book, the definitions of the terms "error" and "adverse event" that we use are the ones adopted by the Institute of Medicine (IOM) in its report *To Err Is Human.*[1]

> An error is defined as the failure of a planned action to be completed as intended (i.e., error of execution) or the use of a wrong plan to achieve an aim (i.e., error of planning).
>
> An adverse event is an injury caused by medical management rather than the underlying condition of the patient. An adverse event attributable to error is a "preventable adverse event."

Negligent adverse events represent a subset of preventable adverse events that satisfy legal criteria used in determining negligence (i.e., whether the care provided failed to meet the standard of care reasonably expected of an average physician qualified to take care of the patient in question).

Another useful concept is that of a "near miss," defined in the QuIC report as "an event or situation that could have resulted in an accident, injury, or illness, but did not, either by chance or through timely intervention."[9] These three concepts can be illustrated in a Venn diagram (fig. 1). As shown in the figure, few adverse events are the result of medical error, and few errors result in adverse events. For example, in one study of medication errors, fully 5 percent of all orders for medication contained errors, but only 1 percent *of these* resulted in an adverse event.[18]

While the IOM definitions seem fairly straightforward, many areas of ambiguity remain. John Banja has provided a hypothetical example that illustrates this dilemma: Dr. Smith is an excellent surgeon who prepares to do an abdominal operation on Mr. Jones. Mr. Jones has had numerous abdominal operations, so Dr. Smith is anticipating a good deal of scarring along with anatomical rearrangement. Despite painstaking care during the surgery, Dr. Smith lacerates Mr. Jones's bowel, causing the need for additional surgery.[19]

Did Dr. Smith commit an error? Clearly the laceration meets the IOM definition of an adverse event, and many would also assume that any unwanted outcome that occurs as part of the management of care must involve an error by someone. Yet this case clearly shows that one needs to be cautious when ascribing accountability for bad outcomes. While Dr. Smith certainly had an obligation to inform Mr. Jones about the potential

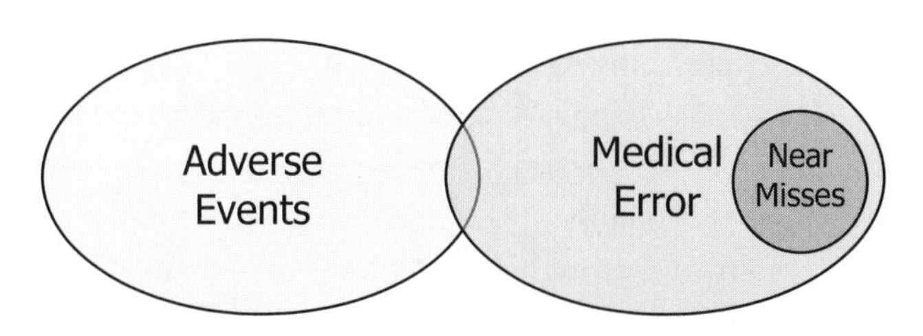

FIGURE 1. The relationship among adverse events, medical error, and near misses

for complications of this type, given the difficulties that could have been anticipated based on the number of previous surgical procedures, this adverse event should rightly be seen as a foreseeable surgical complication, not as a medical error.

For addressing some of the subtlety of cases like these, Albert Wu has offered a more nuanced approach to defining medical error. Similar to the concept of Smith and Forster described above, Wu's suggested definition of error is "an act or an omission with potentially negative consequences for the patient that would have been judged wrong by skilled and knowledgeable peers at the time it occurred."[20] While not as simple as the IOM definition, it better reflects the realities and complexities of modern medicine. Of course, application of this type of definition requires clinical judgment. For cases that fall into a gray zone, determining whether a particular event was an error may require some form of adjudicatory process, such as consideration by a group of impartial experts. Even after careful event analysis, it may sometimes be difficult to know definitively whether an adverse event was due to an error.

Finally, we need to emphasize two very important points about the terminology that we use throughout this book. The first refers to our use of the phrase "adverse events and medical error." This phrase combines all of the concepts illustrated in figure 1. We recognize, of course, that whether an untoward event was an adverse event or a medical error is critically important to everyone involved. Throughout the text, however, we tend to lump these concepts together because, for purposes of disclosure, they are typically handled in the same way.

In the immediate aftermath of an adverse event, clinicians commonly cannot know whether the event was the result of an error. (Exceptions to this include a relatively small set of obvious errors, such as wrong site surgery.) As we discuss in more detail below, initial impressions are almost always incomplete and sometimes completely wrong. But whether or not the incident is ultimately found to be caused by an error, the patient needs to be informed of what has happened and its implications for medical care going forward. This message to the patient is coupled with a commitment that the event will be thoroughly investigated and that the patient will be informed of the results of that inquiry in a timely manner as it unfolds.

The second important point about terminology pertains to our use of the word "disclosure." Both the academic literature on this subject and common usage tend to favor the phrase "disclosure of medical error." Unfortunately, in this context the word "disclosure" conveys a sense that the clinicians are being forced to tell something they would prefer to keep secret. Some countries, like the United Kingdom, have abandoned the term altogether in favor of the broader concept of "being open." ASHRM has addressed this problem as follows in the context of hospital policies:

> When drafting a policy, it is important to determine the language that will be used and the effect of that language. Using the word "disclosure" can often give the impression that the consequences of not having such a policy would indicate "non-disclosure." Instead, using proactive terms such as "communication" may avoid this impression and convey a positive cultural statement.

We agree with this perspective, and in this book we use phrases like "communication about adverse events and medical error" whenever possible but use the language of disclosure whenever it conveys a more accurate description of the issue under discussion.

THREE

A Brief Overview of the Patient Safety Movement

Of course, medical error is not a new problem; it has existed since the first injured or sick patient sought medical care.[20,21] However, the evolution of health care into a complex system, involving multiple specialties, teams of clinicians, different sites of care, and new technologies and medications, has created many more opportunities for medical error and other adverse events.

In the 1980s, some far-thinking health care leaders, including Don Berwick and Paul Bataldan, identified the growing problem in delivering safe, quality care. They experimented with some innovations within their own sphere of influence, looked at the efforts ongoing within other industries (including Toyota, Bell Labs, and NASA), and learned from quality improvement experts such as Deming and Juran.[22] In the 1990s, the prevalence of medical error was brought into even greater focus with the publication of a number of well-respected studies documenting the frequency of such errors.[23]

In 1991, investigators in Boston reported the results of the Harvard Medical Practice Study.[24] This study examined more than 30,000 records from randomly selected acute care hospitals in New York State in 1984. They found that adverse events occurred in 3.7 percent of the hospitalizations and that 28 percent of these were due to negligence, with 14 percent of the adverse events leading to death. This study established the standard by which adverse events could be measured and laid the groundwork for future studies in the United States and other countries to examine the frequency of adverse events and error.[25]

The death of Betsy Lehman, *Boston Globe* reporter and young mother, from a medication overdose at the Dana-Farber Cancer Center, made headlines and raised concern that error could occur even at a world-renowned hospital. In 1996 a number of stakeholders, including the American Medical Association, the American Association for the Advancement of Science, the Veterans Administration, and the Joint Commission on Accreditation of Healthcare Organizations (JCAHO), convened a conference focused on patient safety. In 1998, the President's Advisory Commission on Consumer Protection and Quality in the Health Care Industry released a report that identified medical error as one of the four major challenges facing the industry. These events paved the way for the most significant publication of the 1990s, the report from the Institute of Medicine (IOM).

To Err Is Human: The Sentinel Report

The decision of the Institute of Medicine to undertake the Quality of Health Care in America project, with the participation of a number of health care leaders, including Don Berwick and Lucian Leape, was a watershed in the patient safety movement. The first milestone in this project was the release in 2000 of the sentinel report *To Err Is Human*.[1] The IOM report contained estimates ranging from 44,000 to 98,000 deaths in hospitals each year from medical error, with estimated costs ranging from $17 billion to $29 billion. While the task force acknowledged that medical care is not a risk-free enterprise, it pointed out that the frequency and cost of error in health care far outstripped those found in other high-risk industries.

The 2000 IOM report not only generated widespread concern within the health care industry but also brought the issue of medical error into the public forum, shaking many people's trust in their medical care. The report was notable both for identifying the magnitude of the problem and also for suggesting that the cause of the problem was not the behavior of a few inept practitioners or "bad apples." According to the IOM report, only a small number of medical errors are caused by incompetent practitioners. Most such errors arise from a complex and dynamic interaction of human actors and system factors. Thus, reducing such errors requires a new paradigm for thinking about error—a shift from blaming individuals to understanding the complex causes of error and making systemwide

TABLE 1. Recommendations of the Institute of Medicine, *To Err Is Human,* 2000

- Implement a nationwide system for mandatory reporting of adverse events
- Increase federal and state funding for safety improvement
- Add confidentiality protections for information voluntarily reported
- Adopt nonpunitive systems within institutions to encourage sharing of information about error
- Develop performance standards for safe care
- Increase use of incentives by purchasers to encourage safe practices
- Align payment and liability systems to encourage safety
- Disseminate tools and education to those in the health care field
- Increase patient involvement in the patient safety movement

changes to prevent them. The IOM report also highlighted how the bad apple paradigm had created a culture of silence, one in which health care workers hesitate to report errors to the hospital, making it difficult to analyze and learn from problems in care. The report strongly urged that steps be taken to promote greater transparency in health care and made a number of specific recommendations that became the blueprint for all the subsequent major efforts to improve patient safety (table 1).

The Response to *To Err Is Human*

The response to the 2000 IOM report included actions by individuals and numerous governmental, nonprofit, and grassroots organizations, generating thousands of research documents, reports, Web sites, and programs. We mention a few of them here but also note that one of the most significant achievements of the patient safety movement has been increased access, through professional organizations, research studies, and Web sites (governmental, nonprofit, and private) to a plethora of information about patient safety and quality of care.

Not surprisingly, the literature addressing patient safety increased dramatically after the 2000 IOM report. The number of patient safety publications and research awards grew rapidly, as did publications reporting original research.[26] The IOM itself issued several additional reports as part of its Quality Initiative, including *Crossing the Quality Chasm: A New Health System for the 21st Century*.[27] In this report, the

IOM provided an outline of steps toward a better health care system and also succinctly summarized what patients should expect in the future from health care providers:

- *Information*: You can know what you wish to know, when you wish to know it. Your medical record is yours to keep, to read, and to understand. The rule is: "Nothing about you without you."
- *Safety*: Errors in care will not harm you. You will be safe in the care system.

These dual themes of safety and disclosure run throughout the movement and throughout this book.

As the IOM continued its work, other organizations and individuals also pursued various lines of research, and industry think tanks such as the Rand Corporation, Kaiser Family Foundation, and the Institute for Healthcare Improvement (IHI), directed attention and funds to the effort.[23] One line of research focused on the dimensions of the problem. While most commentators seemed to accept the IOM's conclusion that errors occurred often and were costly, not all agreed with the specific figures contained in the IOM report, and some sought additional data in regard to frequency, cost, and consequences. Some of the studies focused on type of errors—for example, medication errors.[28–32] Others looked at the site of errors, such as errors in intensive care units and outpatient settings.[33–35] Still others examined consequences of errors, such as their correlation with length of stay and mortality.[36] One useful source of data about the frequency of error came from the Medicare program. In 2004, HealthGrades released a study titled *Patient Safety in American Hospitals*, which applied 16 safety indicators developed by the Agency for Healthcare Research and Quality (AHRQ) to three years of Medicare discharge data.[37] The study reported that approximately 1.14 million total patient safety incidents occurred among the 37 million hospitalized Medicare recipients in the years 2000 through 2002, at an excess inpatient cost of $8.54 billion over the three-year period.

Another line of research and analysis pursued after the 2000 IOM report reflected the IOM's call for a more nuanced understanding of the nature of human error—including the complex causes of error and the role of organizational systems. (Authors of one review noted that the subject matter of the patient safety literature changed following the 2000 IOM report, with "organizational culture" replacing "malpractice" as the most frequently addressed topic.)[26] These researchers benefited from existing scholarship devoted to understanding the nature of human error, including James Reason's classic text, *Human Error*, which itself reflected the findings of psychologists and other professionals working in the field.[8] In his text, Reason distinguished active errors, which are made by "front-line performers," from latent errors, which represent breakdowns in the process of care that occur further from the point of service. Reason also popularized the "swiss cheese" model of health care errors, which emphasizes that most errors that cause harm to patients represent the sequential failure of multiple layers of system-level defenses. While latent errors are harder to identify and correct, Reason posited that they pose the biggest challenge to safety in complex, high-technology industries. In March 2000, the *British Medical Journal* devoted an entire issue to patient safety and medical error.[38] The editors noted the impact of the IOM report on "kick-starting" work on this problem in the United States, and while acknowledging that most of the authors represented in the issue were American, they also proudly noted that James Reason was both British and a prominent contributor to that issue of the *BMJ*.

The work of Reason, as well as other insights provided by those studying error in complex organizations, proved useful in the health care arena, and a number of articles and texts began to appear addressing the implications of such research for the patient safety movement. The year 2000 saw the publication of *Error Reduction in Health Care: A Systems Approach to Improving Patient Safety*, containing articles ranging from theoretical discussions of systems' approaches to specific illustrations and suggestions for change.[39] In the foreword, Lucian Leape emphasized the complex causes of error in health care and the need to change significantly how such errors are conceptualized and addressed. In 2004, a collection of articles titled *Achieving Safe and Reliable Healthcare* appeared, focusing on features that define a safe environment—or what is now commonly referred to as a "High Reliability Organization."[40] Many other researchers also contributed to an understanding of how complex organizations work and how they can be made safer.

During this period, the experiences of other industries were offered as examples of successful approaches to error reduction. One such industry was the federal aviation industry, which in 1975 had created an incident-reporting system in response to a fatal crash and a near miss. In order to encourage reporting, the system was made voluntary; those reporting adverse events were deidentified and granted limited immunity, and (for further protection) reports were made to an outside agency.[1] Various programs for quality improvement in other organizations, including Motorola's "Six Sigma Quality" strategy, were also cited. The Six Sigma strategy emphasized collecting, analyzing, and using data to reduce errors or defects to such a low frequency that such an event would constitute a 6 standard deviation difference from the mean functioning of that health care process.[41]

While the theoretical underpinnings of a systems approach to error reduction existed, along with some examples from industry, implementation of such systems in the health care industry was sporadic. While some institutions moved forward in changing their systems,[42] David Marx observed in 2001 that most hospital disciplinary systems continued to unrealistically "prohibit" error, responding to it with censure and disciplinary action.[43] Although the desire for a zero tolerance level for error is understandable, such an emphasis may cause health care personnel to avoid reporting errors, leaving institutions unaware of the extent of such errors within their systems. Marx argued that to improve patient safety the health care culture must be changed so that reporting of errors is encouraged (while certain behaviors, such as "malicious conduct" or "intoxication," remain subject to punitive sanctions). A change in culture is also necessary to encourage clinicians to speak freely with patients and families as well as to share information within their organizations.

The response of the federal government to the IOM report was broad and diverse. Some of the highlights include the following:

- Immediately after the IOM report was released, President Clinton directed the Quality Interagency Coordination (QuIC) Task Force to evaluate the recommendations in *To Err Is Human* and to respond with a strategy to identify prevalent threats to patient safety and reduce medical errors. In its report, QuIC supported each of the IOM recommendations and set forth those steps that the federal government might take to help accomplish them.[9]

- The AHRQ also undertook significant efforts to promote safety, including oversight of a Patient Safety Task Force designed to integrate ongoing research and analysis of medical error. AHRQ also created the National Guidelines Clearinghouse, which maintains a large database of evidence-based clinical practice guidelines for enhancing patient safety, as well as the National Quality Measures Clearinghouse, another source of information for measuring quality.[44]
- In 2005, then Senators Obama and Clinton introduced legislation in Congress designed to encourage clinicians to disclose errors and enter into fair compensation agreements.[45] This act was not passed, but later that year the Congress did pass the Patient Safety and Quality Improvement Act of 2005 (Public Law 109-41),[46] creating Patient Safety Organizations to collect, aggregate, and analyze confidential information reported by health care providers. In response to fears of discovery and use of information in lawsuits, the law included provisions for increased protection under federal law for information voluntary shared. The regulations became effective in January 2009.
- The government also responded to the IOM's recommendation that financial incentives be used to encourage safe, quality care. The Patient Quality Reporting System for providers participating in the Medicare/Medicaid program, initiated in 2006, offered incentives for satisfactory reporting of quality data on specified indicators.[47] There are other financial incentives within the Medicare program for decreasing errors, including regulations stating that the Medicare program will not pay for certain reasonably preventable conditions (nor can hospitals bill patients directly). A number of state Medicaid programs also will not pay for these "never events."

State governments also responded to the recommendation for a nationwide mandatory reporting system for adverse events. In the year 2000, 15 states had mandatory reporting systems, but by 2007, 25 states plus the District of Columbia had mandatory reporting systems focused on patient safety. Most provided general peer review protection for information voluntarily provided, and most featured some public release of the data.

Similarly, whereas in 2000 only one state required disclosure to patients/ families when an adverse event occurred; by 2007, 11 states required such disclosure.[48]

Many private organizations mobilized in response to the IOM report. The following are some of those that resonate within the health care field:

- JCAHO, long an influential standard setter in health care, incorporated patient safety goals into the accreditation process in 2001 and developed a sentinel event database. The JCACO standards continue to emphasize safety and quality, and the organization offers publications, educational programs, and consulting services to assist health care providers achieve these standards (www.jointcommission.org).
- The Institute for Healthcare Improvement is a nonprofit organization with a mission of improving health care worldwide. IHI contributed to the patient safety movement with numerous educational offerings and with programs such as the "100,000 Lives Campaign" and the "5 Million Lives Campaign." IHI's goals are called the "No Needless List" and include "no needless deaths, no needless pain or suffering, no helplessness in those served or serving, no unwanted waiting, no waste, and no one left out" (www.IHI.org).
- The National Quality Forum (NQF), a private organization whose members include public and private employers, unions, insurers, health systems, providers, vendors, consumer organizations, and accrediting bodies, was also responsive to the need for change. In 2003, NQF endorsed 30 "safe practices" for reducing error and improving care. Through 2008, NQF has endorsed more than 500 measures, indicators, practices and products. It describes its endorsement as the "gold standard" for measuring health care quality (www.qualityforum.org).
- Another private group, the Leapfrog Group for Patient Safety, formed in 1989 by a consortium of large employers committed to using their purchasing power to influence the quality and affordability of health care, exercised its influence to encourage the public reporting of outcomes. The Leapfrog Group issues

hospital quality ratings and works to reward providers for improving the safety, quality, and affordability of care (www.leapgfroggroup.org).

- The American Society of Healthcare Risk Management (ASHRM), founded in 1980, is another private group that has been actively involved in the patient safety movement since its inception. Its activities include advocacy, education, research, and publication, including key monographs on patient safety and disclosure of adverse events to patients (www.ashrm.org).

Individual patients and clinicians have also spoken out about their experiences with adverse events and formed support and advocacy groups. Among these are the following:

- Medically Induced Trauma Support Services (MITSS) is an organization that was founded by a patient and a clinician who discovered that open communication helped them recover and heal from the pain caused by an adverse outcome. MITSS continues to "support healing and support hope" among patients, families, and clinicians who have experienced an adverse medical event (www.mits.org).
- The organization "SorryWorks!" was founded by an individual whose brother died as a result of an adverse event (a successful law suit was brought by the family). Doug Wojciezak was struck by the fact that until the lawsuit was over, no one apologized to the family, and the providers never accepted fault. The coalition he founded, which includes ethicists, consumers, and others active in the patient safety movement, is committed to the belief that a patient-focused, open, and compassionate response to adverse events will not only reduce distress among patients, families, and clinicians but will also reduce the frequency with which patients bring legal actions against their providers. The coalition offers training sessions, videos, and written material, including a handbook outlining its philosophy and a recommended disclosure program (www.sorryworks.net).

The activities listed above are far from a complete accounting of the response stimulated by the revelations of the 2000 report from the Institute of Medicine, but they provide a flavor of the initiatives seen at the federal, state, and private levels.

After *To Err Is Human*: Progress, or Not?

During the years following publication of *To Err Is Human,* numerous efforts were undertaken to reduce the incidence of medical error. Yet despite these steps, many believed that the efforts had fallen short of the goals established by the IOM and that the incidence of errors remains unacceptably high.

For example, in the first few years after the IOM report, surveys indicated that patients continued to experience medical error at a high rate. In one study from 2001, 34 percent of those surveyed reported that they or a member of their family had experienced a medical error.[49] In 2002, another study indicated that 42 percent of the public surveyed reported such errors and 35 percent of physicians did as well.[50] In 2004, a survey by the Kaiser Family Foundation indicated that a little more than one-third of those surveyed reported personal or family experiences of error. Forty percent of those surveyed thought that the quality of care had declined over the previous three years, and 48 percent said they were concerned about the safety of health care.[51]

General measurements of safety in health care also suggested that medical errors remained a significant problem. For each of the years 2000, 2001, and 2002, HealthGrades estimated 195,000 hospital deaths due to potentially preventable errors.[52] In 2003, AHRQ issued the first national governmental report on health care quality, concluding that despite significant progress in improving quality and safety of care in a number of key areas, little progress had been made in other areas and quality of care varied significantly across sites.[53]

HealthGrades has continued to evaluate patient safety through its annual reports. In 2008, it released another study using Medicare data from 2004 to 2006. This study found a decrease in all-cause mortality rates among patients who experienced adverse events, and improvement was seen in a majority of patient safety indicators. However, the data also found more than a million patient safety incidents occurring in about 40 million hospitalizations, with $8.8 billion in excess costs.[54]

In trying to sum up the first five years after publication of the IOM report, commentators generally agreed that while many positive steps had been taken, much more remained to be done.[55–58] Some of the improvements cited included increased funding for AHRQ and positive responses to new JCAHO safety goals. Despite these steps, progress was slow, and the frequency of medical errors remained high. The frequency of high profile medical errors such as wrong site surgeries appeared not to have changed, despite large-scale campaigns by JCAHO and others to reduce these events. It was also noted that the views of physicians, the public, and safety experts were not always consonant and that broader cultural changes were necessary to encourage the sharing of information about errors.

In the years following the fifth anniversary of the IOM report, the patient safety movement continued to grow rapidly and achieve greater integration with the general movement toward enhanced quality of care. Numerous and varied efforts to improve patient safety and quality continued. One important focus of this work was on refining standards or indicators for safety and quality. Some of the accomplishments are as follows:

- Beginning in 2003, AHRQ has made available a set of patient safety indicators to be used by institutions to identify potential adverse events and to measure and compare performance across institutions. According to AHQR, information about the indicators can be gathered from readily available hospital administrative data. AHRQ has used these indicators in its annual National Healthcare Quality Reports. In general, these reports have indicated that gains continue to be made in health care safety and quality. However, each report has also included the observation that progress is, in some cases, halting. In the 2007 report, AHRQ attempted to summarize what progress had been made and what challenges remain for achieving desired quality and safety goals. It concluded that (1) health care quality continues to improve, but at a slower rate, (2) variations in health care quality have decreased in some but not all measures, and (3) the safety of health care has improved since 2000, but more needs to be done.[59]

- AHRQ has also developed a survey for use by hospitals in determining whether their institution has a culture of safety. The results reflect self-reporting and are focused on certain areas considered key to a culture of patient safety. The results for 2007, 2008, and 2009 are quite similar; those for 2009 are summarized in figure 2. Interestingly, the category in the survey with the second-to-lowest positive response is that reflecting staff's view as to whether their culture has a nonpunitive response to error, despite the fact that the creation of a nonpunitive environment has been considered key to creating a culture of safety.
- The National Quality Forum has also been active in promulgating and refining safety standards and measures since 1999. In 2006 NQF released a list of "serious reportable events" that it believed should never happen. These became well known throughout medicine as "never events." The Leapfrog Group subsequently offered public recognition to hospitals that agreed that if a "never event" were to occur, they would apologize, report the event to a safety organization, perform a root cause analysis, and waive costs directly related to the event.
- AHRQ has collaborated with the National Association of Children's Hospitals and Related Institutions (NACHRI) to develop more targeted measures of quality. NACHRI has initiated a multiyear project focused on preventing a specific type of adverse event (catheter-associated blood stream infections [CABSIs] in pediatric intensive care units). NACHRI reported that, in the first year, participating institutions experienced a 43 percent decrease in CABSI events; prevented an estimated 275 infections and an estimated 40 deaths; and realized a $9 million cost savings.

Another focused area for potential safety improvements is residency practice—in particular, the number of hours that residents work. Triggered in part by the well-publicized case of Libby Zion, who died in a New York Hospital Emergency Department in 1984, various studies have attempted to determine whether residents' schedules have an impact on

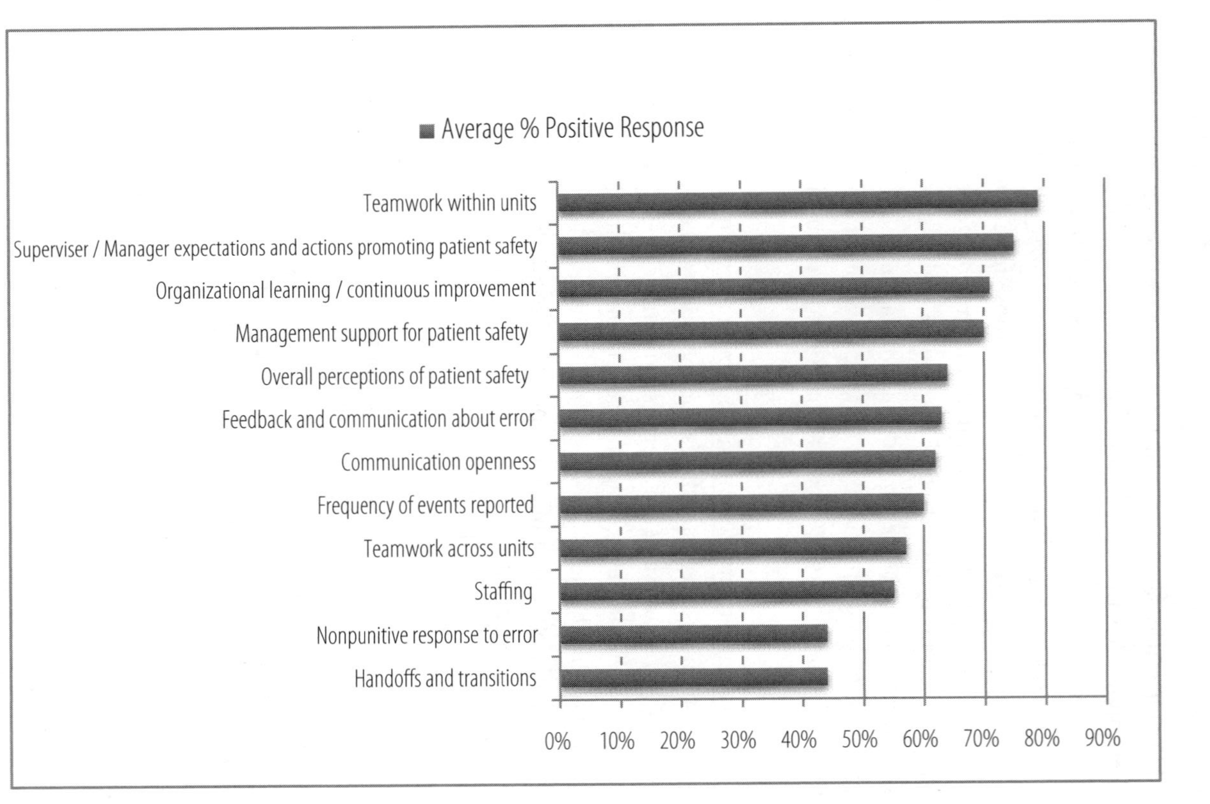

FIGURE 2. Hospital Survey on Patient Safety Culture, 2009 Comparative Database Report. *Source:* AHRQ Publication No. 09-0030, April 2009. Agency for Healthcare Research and Quality, Rockville, MD. Used with permission. http://www.ahrq.gov/qual/patientsafetyculture/

patient safety (including the Bell Commission Report formed after Zion's death). Based on increased knowledge about the consequences of sleep deprivation (accompanied by the increase in acuity and intensity of hospital care provided by residents), the Accreditation Council on Graduate Medical Education (ACGME) instituted a limit on residents' work hours in 2003. Controversy still exists as to the effects of such limitations, and the ACGME is looking more broadly at ways in which medical education can evolve to meet the challenge of providing safe care while preserving essential elements of the educational process for young physicians.[60]

There are, of course, many other examples of efforts to improve safety and quality of care over the years from 1999 to 2008. An optimistic view of the progress that has resulted from these efforts was expressed by Lucian Leape, one of the leaders in the patient safety movement, who noted in 2007 that achieving zero adverse events may be a realistic goal.[61] Indeed, Peter Pronovost and colleagues reported on an intervention to decrease catheter-related bloodstream infections in the ICU, demonstrating a dramatic reduction in this complication to rates near zero.[62] In addition to dramatic demonstration projects like this, Leape pointed to the increased use of simulation in training, more sophisticated ways of identifying adverse events, national efforts to ensure physician competency, recognition of the need to disclose errors, and the decision of insurers to cease payment for "never events" as factors that could lead to the elimination of adverse events. Some health care organizations have joined Leape in taking up the challenge for elimination of all adverse events.[63]

Yet others have questioned the wisdom of aspiring to eliminate all adverse events. In a provocative editorial entitled "Is Zero the Ideal Death Rate?" Thomas Lee and colleagues warn about the risk of unintended consequences. They discuss the example of balloon valvuloplasty for congenital aortic stenosis. If the only outcome is safety, they argue, cardiologists will be strongly motivated to use the smallest balloon possible, since this will result in the lowest complication rate. But the price of increasing safety in this instance is decreased efficacy—smaller balloons are less effective at relieving the obstruction and increase the need for additional procedures in the future. In short, focusing only on safety distorts the clinicians' decision-making process and prevents that physician from making the best choice in terms of balancing the risks and benefits of the procedure.[64]

Aside from steering clinicians away from the best medical decisions for their patients, the drive for perfection also demonstrates some of the rhetorical pitfalls that come along with success. The notion of "zero adverse events" can itself be an impediment to improvement because (1) most adverse events are not the result of error, (2) not all adverse events are preventable, (3) no human endeavor is free from error, and (4) advocating "zero adverse events" may inhibit the willingness of clinicians to acknowledge errors when they occur, thus undercutting a key feature of the patient safety movement. According to Dr. Leape, these calls for perfection have been articulated for their inspirational and motivational value and are not intended literally.[65] Even so, while there may be disagreement about whether the "right" goal is "zero," there is little disagreement about the importance of efforts to reduce the number of mistakes causing death, including efforts to increase transparency and communication as fundamental to achieving safer care.

FOUR

Communicating about Adverse Events and Medical Error

Lucian Leape has championed the importance of disclosure and apology on the solid ethical grounds that it is "the right thing to do," and indeed, that should be sufficient. However, in a world in which clinicians fear that a single error could bring ruin to their professional reputations and financial devastation to them and their families, this admonition to take the moral highroad can at times prove to be a hard sell. The emergence of data showing that the ethically correct action may also be aligned with the clinicians' best interest has therefore been welcomed as an opportunity to transform practice and institutional culture. In this chapter we briefly review the development of disclosure and apology in medicine over the past few decades and describe how views on these complex issues have evolved.

Needs and Desires of Patients and Families

Patients and their families overwhelmingly desire full and honest communication with their providers following adverse outcomes.[15,66–68] In many cases, this desire for disclosure extends to minor errors[12,69] and, in some cases, even "near misses."[15,70,71] Honesty is seen as an inherent feature of the patient-physician relationship, and failure to disclose may be considered a breach of trust that adversely affects the relationship.[72] Silence or evasion may increase patients' stress; providing limited information to patients may be construed as detachment and may signal, to patients, a withdrawal from the patient-physician relationship.[15,73]

The type of information desired by patient and families is also fairly clear. They want to know what happened—an explanation of the adverse event itself—and also why it happened. They want to know what is going to be done to prevent a future recurrence. In addition, patients want to be asked about their needs—medical, emotional, and financial.[15,70,72] While experiencing an adverse event has been shown to cause physical, emotional, and financial trauma, patients and families report less trauma if they have experienced "good" communication with their clinicians.[74,75] There is also evidence that when patients suffer injury caused by an adverse event, they seek validation of, and compassion for, their suffering; failure to acknowledge and empathize with their pain can be perceived an additional injury. When a clear error has occurred, patients want some expression of regret and an appropriate apology. Certainly in cases of clear error, the failure to acknowledge the patient's injury, accept responsibility appropriately, and apologize may prevent the patient and family from being able to forgive the clinician's mistake and thus prevent the restoration of the clinician-patient relationship.[76,77]

It is not only the content of the communication that is important but also the way in which the communication is handled; for example, respectful and caring communication, attention to the needs of the patient, and an apology have been found helpful in maintaining patients' relationships with their caregivers. Good communication has also been found to increase the likelihood that the patient perceives the event as a mistake rather than a demonstration of incompetence. One study, using hypothetical cases, showed that patients' responses to adverse events were adversely influenced not only by the seriousness of the health consequences but also by a lack of staff responsiveness and failure to disclose. While health outcomes were an important factor in the patients' responses, slow and ineffective handling of errors increased patients' negative reactions regardless of the level of seriousness of the outcome.[78] In addition, research has demonstrated that patients and families respond negatively to the perception that clinicians are avoiding accountability or trying to prevent a lawsuit or providing information only in response to patient or family demands.[69,79–83]

Lack of communication not only fails to meet patient's immediate needs, but may also influence their future interactions with the health care system. One study has shown that experiencing medical error may influ-

TABLE 2. Patient and Physician Attitudes about Medical Error Disclosure

Focus Group Themes	Patients' Attitudes	Physicians' Attitudes
Definition of error	Broad: includes deviations from the standard of care, some nonpreventable adverse events, poor service quality, and deficient interpersonal skills of practitioners	Narrow: deviations from accepted standard of care only
What errors to disclose	All errors that cause harm	Errors that cause harm, except when harm is trivial, patient cannot understand error, or patient does not want to know about error
Disclose near misses?	Mixed	No
What information to disclose about error	Tell everything	Choose words carefully
How to disclose error	Truthfully and compassionately	Truthfully, objectively, and professionally
Role of apology	Desirable	Concerned that apology creates a legal liability
Emotional impact of error	Upset, angry, scared	Upset that patient was harmed and about how error could impact career

Source: Gallagher TH, Waterman AD, Ebers AG, Fraser VJ, Levinson W. Patients' and physicians' attitudes regarding the disclosure of medical errors. *JAMA*. 2003;289: 1001–1007.

ence patients not to return to the health care provider.[14] In another study, patients reported feeling anger and a lack of trust after experiencing an adverse event, and some of them indicated they would avoid seeking health care services in the future.[16] Table 2 summarizes a comparison of the attitudes of patients with those of physicians about the disclosure of medical error.

Ethical Norms Regarding Disclosure of Error

Greater communication and transparency with respect to adverse events is in accord with the widespread consensus that disclosure of information to patients and families after an adverse event is an ethical obligation.

This consensus is supported by standard theories, methods, and reasoning in the field of clinical ethics.[10]

One basis for the duty to disclose all outcomes of care (including adverse outcomes) is the fiduciary nature of the physician's relationship with the patient, which obligates the physician to be trustworthy and to act in the patient's best interests.[10,84] Another basis is the principle of respect for persons, which requires acting in a way that acknowledges the worth and dignity of the patient and abjures any form of deception. The principle of autonomy (self-determination) and the doctrine of informed consent also require a physician to disclose all information relevant to the patient's decision making.[20,85] Another principle supporting full disclosure after an adverse event is justice: patients who suffer damages from medical error should be compensated for these harms. To seek just compensation, they need to know what happened. Full disclosure, and apology when appropriate, also reflect the values of truth telling and compassion and the virtues of honesty, trustworthiness, and courage. To respond ethically to an error, the clinician must be honest and humble enough to disclose the mistake; apologize to those who have been affected; and make amends when possible.[11]

The principle of consequentialism, which involves a weighing of the benefits and harms of an action, also supports disclosure. This principle suggests that disclosure can benefit the patient in that it contributes to the patient's understanding and ability to make an informed decision. It provides consolation to the patient in the form of knowledge that steps are being taken to avoid similar events in the future. Honest disclosure, and apology when appropriate, also help to maintain the integrity of clinicians and to alleviate their sense of guilt. Failure to disclosure, in contrast, involves deceit and elevates professional interests over the interests of patients, thereby undermining public trust in medicine.

Narrative ethics also makes a powerful contribution to an understanding of the effects of adverse events on patients, families, and clinicians. Through their stories, patients and families have communicated the detrimental effects of nondisclosure and emotional withdrawal by clinicians. They have reported feelings of abandonment, lost of trust, grief, and anger.[74,86,87] Clinicians, through their stories, have told of the negative effect on them of failure to disclose and to empathize or apologize to their patients. They have reported feelings of isolation, inadequacy, depression, and grief.[3,88,89]

A number of scholars have applied knowledge and experiences from other fields, such as religious study, psychology, sociology, and political science, to the ethical issues raised by the occurrence of adverse events in medicine. Nancy Berlinger, a scholar who approaches the issues in the context of religious traditions, describes the aftermath of medical harm as a process that extends from error through disclosure, apology, and repentance to forgiveness. (She notes that while use of the term "forgiveness" may seem to suggest a religious belief, the concept has actually "permeated secular culture in the West" for a long time.)[74] In his work on apology, Aaron Lazare draws on studies in psychology as well as sociology and, using examples ranging from apologies by individuals to apologies by governments, argues for the importance of disclosure and apology.[75]

Although all the ethical "vectors" described above point in the direction of disclosure, one consistent feature of all ethical analysis is that ethical principles may come into conflict. For example, the ethical duty to disclose may come into conflict with the ethical duty of nonmaleficence (the duty not to harm). In a situation in which an error was of no (or minimal) consequence to the patient, disclosure might only serve to shake the patient's confidence in the care being given and result in increased and needless anxiety. As another example, some have observed that literally hundreds of events do not go perfectly in every hospital every day. If medical culture were to change such that clinicians felt an obligation to disclose all of these events, an enormous amount of time would have to be devoted to these disclosure conversations, taking valuable time away from other essential aspects of care. They worry that such a culture could have the perverse and unintended consequence of actually decreasing the overall quality of care.

Toward the end of the book, we address some of these concerns when we discuss a broad spectrum of cases, and we consider the question of whether and when disclosure is not ethically required. In this regard, however, it is extremely important to remember that the prevailing culture still tends to look for any excuse to justify nondisclosure, and we must resist any tendency to emphasize ethical loopholes that make it easier for clinicians to justify nondisclosure in situations in which most would agree it is ethically required. While there are certainly some situations where nondisclosure is the right thing to do, the threshold for reaching this decision must be set fairly high.

Professional Ethical Standards

The ethical norms with regard to disclosure have been translated into concrete professional ethical standards, providing additional impetus for greater transparency after adverse events. For example, the American Medical Association states that it is a "fundamental ethical requirement" that a physician deal honestly and openly with patients at all times. Specifically, when a patient suffers medical complications possibly caused by the physician's mistake or judgment, the physician is required to inform the patient of all the facts necessary to ensure that the patient understands what has occurred. Concerns about legal liability should not affect the physician's disclosure.[90] The American Nurses Association also supports disclosure, noting that nurses have a duty not to be involved in or condone attempts to cover up an error or attempts to fix blame without correcting conditions leading to the problem. Nurses also are expected to report errors in accordance with institutional policies and to ensure responsible disclosure to patients.[91] The American College of Physicians states that "physicians should disclose to patients information about procedural or judgment errors made in the course of care if such information is material to the patient's well-being."[92]

Other physician groups have similar professional standards. Several have adopted the document entitled "Medical Professionalism in the New Millennium: A Physician Charter," which contains a commitment that whenever patients are injured through medical care, the patient should be promptly informed; failure to disclose seriously compromises the patient's, and society's, trust.[93] The American College of Surgeons includes within its Code of Professional Conduct recognition of the value of the trust the patient has in the physician. Accordingly, surgeons should accept responsibility for fully disclosing adverse events and medical errors.[94]

Benefits of Disclosure

We have seen that Lucian Leape's admonition that disclosure is "the right thing to do" is supported by ethical analysis and enshrined in professional standards. Furthermore, in an era in which improving and enhancing "patient-centered care" has become a virtual litmus test for any proposed changes in our health care system, it is hard to imagine any reform that has the potential to integrate patients more powerfully into their own care than a commitment to sharing knowledge with them about adverse events and errors. In addition to these considerations, however, there is a growing body of empirical evidence showing that disclosure offers other substantial benefits to patients and clinicians alike, as summarized in table 3.

One of the most compelling benefits of transparency and disclosure in the wake of adverse events is the potential for enhancing patient safety.[95,96] While there may be some differences in estimates as to the number of patients injured in the course of medical care, there is little disagreement that the figure needs to be reduced. To effect such a change, the sources and/or causes of such events must be known and analyzed so that corrective actions can be taken. Open communication has been called "the cornerstone" of the patient safety movement.[97] To promote such communication, the patient safety movement is working to replace a culture of "shame and blame," or "deny and defend," with a culture of transparency and compassion for patients and clinicians alike.[42]

TABLE 3. The Benefits of Disclosure

- Sharing information improves patient safety and reduces the frequency, cost, and patient suffering associated with adverse events
- Disclosure decreases patient frustration and anger over lack of information and perceived lack of empathy from caregivers
- Disclosure mitigates clinician distress over broken relationships with patients and facilitates peer support
- Disclosure honors the consensus that ethics and professional responsibilities require honest and empathic communications about adverse events
- Disclosure alleviates the concern, even among lawyers and risk managers, that inadequate communication actually increases legal exposure

In addition to these patient-centered benefits, improving safety and effectiveness is expected to reduce the cost of health care. Thus, those individuals and organizations who are deeply concerned about the cost of health care in the United States, and its implications for access to care, provide further support for the transparency that is so crucial to improving care, as do public and private insurers who are no longer willing to pay for care characterized as "never events."

The Disclosure Gap

Despite these compelling rationales in favor of disclosure, empirical studies as well as personal narratives of patients and clinicians reveal a culture in which communication of potentially incriminating information has traditionally been avoided entirely or greatly circumscribed. Commonly, the facts surrounding an adverse event were shared, if at all, only among a few professional colleagues. They were rarely discussed with patients and families. While this tradition of nondisclosure may be slowly changing, most evidence suggests that disclosure is the exception rather than the norm, even in the present.

The practice of nondisclosure was noted in many studies, both before and after the 2000 IOM report. For example, Wu and colleagues found that medical errors are common but physician disclosure of such errors is not.[98] Based on a review of the literature, Mazor and her colleagues noted that while physicians generally express support of disclosure, in responding to specific scenarios and questions they report a fairly high percentage of cases in which they would not disclose.[76]

Gallagher and colleagues have extensively studied attitudes and practices of clinicians regarding disclosure. Their research shows that as many as 98 percent of physicians agree that serious errors should be disclosed to patients and families.[99,100] At the same time, clinicians have many reservations about disclosure of error, especially in cases in which they believe the harm was not significant or in which the patient would not otherwise know about the error. In one study, for example, more than 2,500 medical and surgical physicians in the United States and Canada were presented with hypothetical scenarios, all of which were regarded by the physicians as representing a serious error.[100] The study found that fewer than half of the physicians would use the word "error" in their conversation with the patient, and only 33 percent would offer an explicit apology, as in "I am so sorry that you were harmed by this error." Furthermore, physicians would disclose less information about errors that the patient would not be aware of compared with errors that were more apparent to the patient. Surgical physicians and medical physicians were also noted to take significantly different approaches to disclosure.

Other research confirms that physicians' practices may not match their stated ideals. Kaldjian and colleagues have shown, for example, that the number of disclosure conversations reported by clinicians is far smaller than what one would expect based on the calculated incidence of harm-causing errors.[101,102]

In a hypothetical study of this issue, Chan and colleagues posed hypothetical cases to a sample of surgeons. One of them, for example, was: "You performed a splenectomy on Mr. Smith, a 60-year-old obese gentleman. On post-operative day one, Mr. Smith develops a low-grade fever and a dry cough. A chest x-ray is ordered and . . . shows a surgical sponge in the left upper quadrant of the abdomen. You remember that the sponge count was correct at the end of the operation. However, you also remember that you were significantly behind schedule that day and do not recall performing your usual final check of the surgical site for foreign bodies."[103]

The surgeons were asked how they would explain this incident to the patient and then were videotaped disclosing the error to standardized patients. Overall, the surgeons used the word "error" or "mistake" in only 57 percent of disclosure conversations, instead using words like "problem" or "complication," without suggesting that the incident was preventable. Overall, they took responsibility for the error in 65 percent of the encounters and offered a verbal apology in 47 percent. In the surgical sponge case described above, they frequently implicated the nursing staff by emphasizing the error in the sponge count.

In another study, Fein and colleagues found that while most clinicians agreed that they would disclose an error, the majority of the respondents engaged in one of the following types of disclosure: (1) "partial" disclosure, which included most but not all of the elements desired by patients; (2) "connect the dots" disclosure, which required the patient to make the link between error and harm; (3) "misleading" disclosure, which left the impression that the outcome was a result of the patient's condition; (4) "deferring" disclosure, which hedged the connection known to exist between error and outcome and suggested other possible explanations to be pursued; and (5) nondisclosure. The study showed that the professionals' view of disclosure was complex and reflected competing values such as disclosure versus self-protection.[104]

Many physicians report that their reticence to disclose is based primarily on fear of litigation—that they would like to express regret, even apologize, but fear such expressions would be seen as an admission of liability.[15,105] This issue was explored by Gallagher and colleagues in a comparison of physicians in the United States and Canada.[100] The results showed that the attitudes and practices of physicians in the two countries regarding disclosure of medical error were quite similar despite the different malpractice systems. While U.S. physicians did report higher estimates of the likelihood of malpractice lawsuits and Canadian physicians were somewhat more supportive of disclosing serious errors, the malpractice environment was not the overwhelming determinant of physicians' attitudes. This research suggests that other factors, such as fear for one's professional reputation, personal guilt, or professional shame, may be more important than malpractice concerns in explaining the reluctance of physicians to disclose medical error.

Personal narratives also provide evidence that patients are often not told about medical errors or are given only a limited amount of information. *Wall of Silence: The Untold Story of the Medical Mistakes That Kill and Injure Millions of Americans,* which appeared several years after the publication of the IOM report, presents a series of dramatic stories collected from patients and families who experienced medical error.[87] In many cases, the patients and families report not being given much—or any—information about what happened, not receiving any acknowledgment of responsibility by providers, and not hearing any expressions of regret or sorrow. Other patients and families have written of their bewilderment, frustration, and anger over the lack of information about, and lack of empathy for, injury suffered from medical error. For example, in her memoir, Sandra Gilbert, poet and scholar, described the trauma that she and her family suffered as a result of her husband's death due to medical error. She notes that their suffering was exacerbated by the silence of the caregivers and the hospital in which he died.[106] The film *When Things*

Go Wrong, which we use in our teaching, offers comments by patients and families who have experienced medical error, including in some cases frank and painful criticism of the lack of information and compassion such patients and families received.[86]

Various reasons have been posited for the wall of silence. One explanation is that key characteristics of the medical culture contribute to a reluctance to disclose information about adverse events. One of these characteristics has been described as a preoccupation with perfection, which contributes to the belief that clinicians who have been properly trained and act in good faith do not make mistakes.[10] The view of the physician as infallible is comforting to a vulnerable patient and also to the physician, who must live up to his or her role as healer. It also reinforces and justifies a physician's position of authority and aura of certainty. Given what has been called the "fantasy of perfection,"[107] physicians are not prepared to deal with their mistakes; they hide them from themselves, their patients, and their colleagues. When they do acknowledge a personal failing, they may suffer strong feelings of guilt, remorse, and inadequacy.[3]

One medical ethicist has suggested that there may be psychological bases for this model of perfection. In his text *Medical Errors and Medical Narcissism*, Banja posits a type of narcissism that may be fostered by medical training and practice.[84] The author suggests that "medical narcissists" are characterized by emotional guardedness, lack of empathy, and controlling behaviors. Because their work affirms their worth, if faced with the possibility of error, they may rationalize or resort to emotional detachment as a form of self-protection. Banja's book highlights how easy it can be for clinicians to focus primarily on how the error affects them personally, rather than approaching disclosure as a fundamentally patient-centered activity.

Another feature of the medical culture identified as contributing to nondisclosure is the nature of medical education and the medical profession. The training of medical professionals takes place in a structured, hierarchical system, within which trainees must perform to the satisfaction of their superiors. In medical training, this may translate into a need to project confidence, even in the face of uncertainty, and appear objective, even in situations that engender confusion and distress. Trainees are socialized early to utilize certain coping mechanisms in the face of error, such as denial, discounting, and distancing.[108,109] Acknowledging vulnerability and the possibility of mistakes is not encouraged or rewarded. In addition, competition is often keen among peers, providing another incentive for projecting strength and detachment.[4]

Medical education and training has done a poor job of addressing how to communicate with patients and families about adverse events.[102,110] When trainees enter practice, they typically find themselves in hierarchical settings, with chiefs of staff or chief medical officers and department heads or chairs who exert substantial influence over their futures. Any tendency developed during training to rationalize or deny error may be reinforced.

Research on physician attitudes has shown that physicians feel poorly prepared in general for communicating effectively with patients and families.[15,21,102,111] Communicating about adverse events and medical errors is particularly difficult because it is fraught with emotion and legal concerns. Physicians are unsure as to what to say and how and when to say it.[99] While some trainees and new practitioners find individual mentors who are skilled at such conversations, many do not. Given the traditional culture of silence about adverse events, few senior clinicians may be able to serve as role models for open and empathic communication. Physicians are likely, in fact, to observe that the accepted practice is to deny or avoid discussion of errors.[108]

As is characteristic of many professions, the practice of medicine has a long tradition of self-control and self-regulation, based in part on the belief that only members of the profession can judge other practitioners. Evaluating the quality of care provided in a clinical setting therefore generally falls to other clinicians. Peer review meetings have traditionally been highly confidential and tightly controlled. The idea of open discussions of professional practices, and particularly possible errors in practice, runs counter to this cultural bias.

One forum that presents an opportunity for change is the traditional "Morbidity and Mortality" conference, or "M&M."[31,112,113] These conferences are highly structured—even ritualized—but they famously provide a setting where clinicians are expected to be open and nondefensive in scrutinizing how their errors may have played a role in the adverse outcomes under discussion. Sometimes even the most senior and experienced staff will be particularly forthcoming about their errors in technique and judgment, providing more junior colleagues with role models of humility and honesty. This atmosphere of candor is tolerated and encouraged, at least in part, by the fact that attendance at these meetings is strictly controlled and limited to those in the close fraternity of the clinical department, and a code of confidentiality is strictly enforced.[4] While M&Ms have traditionally not addressed disclosure to the patient, recently some programs have begun to include this element in their case review, addressing not only whether disclosure occurred but also the nature of the information that was included in the discussion, whether the conversation with the patient went well, and what might have been done to make it go better.

The Effect of Disclosure on Clinicians

While most attention to medical error has, appropriately, been focused on the suffering of patients and families, medical error can also be emotionally traumatic for clinicians. Lucian Leape has referred to clinicians as the "second victims" of medical error. In one study, when attending physicians were asked about the impact of medical errors on their lives, 42 percent noted an impact on their job satisfaction, 47 percent on their confidence in their ability as a physician, and 40 percent on their ability to sleep.[111] Clinicians have reported emotions ranging from shame, anguish, and sadness to panic, remorse, and self-doubt.[3,10,88,114] Clinicians may have difficulty finding appropriate outlets for their emotions, and many express the desire that their suffering be acknowledged and their emotional needs supported.[89,115]

One reason posited for clinicians' suffering after an adverse event is that the traditional silence and lack of open communication with patients are inconsistent with clinicians' perceptions of their moral duty to disclose. This dissonance contributes to their moral distress. Evidence suggests that some physicians feel a desire, based on their relationship with the patient, to communicate openly about adverse events and to express their empathy and sadness over a patient's (or family's) suffering.[15,98,102] Physicians have reported frustration at being advised by risk management and legal advisers to not talk openly with patients and families.[3,88]

Disclosure of medical error may therefore be healing not only for patients but also for clinicians. In one study, two-thirds of the clinicians responding to a survey expressed the belief that disclosing medical error to their patient would help alleviate their feelings of guilt.[102] In another study, 74 percent of physicians and surgeons who had disclosed serious error reported experiencing relief.[100] Some have suggested that in addition to disclosure, an authentic expression of remorse is ethically right and also potentially healing for both patient and physician.[116] Others have used lessons from a religious framework to explore ways in which clinicians can find resolution after medical error. They find the following "commonalities" among religious traditions: (1) breaches that occur in a relationship may lead to a sense of "brokenness" felt by both parties; (2) the person who commits harm has a moral obligation to recognize, apologize, and make amends; (3) the person harmed has an obligation to accept atonement and give forgiveness.[74]

Recently, more attention has been focused on the needs of these "second victims." One support organization, Medically Induced Trauma Support Services (MITSS), was formed in Boston several years ago by an anesthesiologist and his patient after a near fatal drug error during a routine anesthetic. The anesthesiologist had initially been advised against having any communication with the patient, but after several months he went against legal advice and contacted her. Over time, reconciliation occurred, with the creation of an organization to provide support services to both clinicians and patients suffering from the consequences of medical error.

The Effect of Disclosure on Malpractice Litigation

As noted above, one of the most commonly cited reasons for the reluctance of professionals to disclose medical error is fear of litigation.[15,105,117] Litigation carries with it the threat of financial loss, public criticism, loss of reputation, and emotional distress.

The basis for this fear lies in the way in which compensation from medical harm can be recovered in the United States. Under our tort system, patients who experience harm from medical error can generally obtain compensation only by going to court and proving negligence (that is, by showing the existence of a duty owed to the patient by the practitioner, the existence of a standard of care required of one with such a duty, the harm suffered by the patient, and "causation"—that is, a showing that the harm resulted from the breach of the standard of care).[118,119] Although there has been some evolution in the tort system in response to social change, the system continues to operate primarily on the basis of individual responsibility and is not well adapted to deal with injury caused by the complex interactions of individuals and systems. The very conduct of a trial is adversarial and inevitably contains elements of blame and punishment.[120]

The current system has also been criticized for a lack of congruence between actual negligence and successful outcomes in lawsuits; the awarding of large verdicts by juries, which seem to some practitioners to be evidence of economic motives for lawsuits; and the inevitable "hindsight bias" of malpractice actions. Thus, to many practitioners, the system does not seem fair: those patients who win compensation through the court may not have experienced negligence, and many who have experienced negligence are not rewarded through the court system.[121–123]

In addition to the general limitations of the tort system, there is one particular element of a negligence case that may affect a provider's willingness to disclose information to the patient or family. In establishing the standard of care, and also causation, the patient may introduce comments made by the physician or other provider—such as expressions of responsibility, regret, or apology. Because such expressions might be used to support the claim of negligence, risk managers, lawyers, and insurers may counsel practitioners not to talk to patients or their families about the event. It has been posited that there is even some risk (although not great) that a physician could lose malpractice coverage for making such comments, potentially in violation of the so-called cooperation clauses found in many insurance policies.[124] The issue of apology as a part of communication about adverse events and medical error is discussed in greater detail below.

The big question, then, is what would be the overall impact of the adoption of widespread open disclosure practices on malpractice litigation? At this point, the answer is not clear, with varying lines of evidence pointing in opposite directions.

At one end of the spectrum are some data indicating that malpractice costs may remain stable or even be reduced by the adoption of open disclosure policies. For example, there is evidence that open disclosure and a positive relationship with a patient and family may reduce the chances of a lawsuit and that failure to disclose (often seen as attempts to cover up) may increase the likelihood of a suit.[20,81,125–127] Some plaintiffs' lawyers report that their evaluation of the chance of successful litigation is influenced by the clinician's attitude and behavior. If the clinician can be seen as arrogant, unsympathetic, or deceptive, the plaintiff's chance of success is higher. As the president of the South Carolina Trial Association stated in testimony before the South Carolina Senate, "I would never introduce a doctor's apology in court. It is my job to make a doctor look bad in front of a jury, and telling the jury the doctor apologized and tried to do the right thing kills my case."[128]

Similar conclusions were drawn from research involving mock trials. In one study, where two juries were asked to set damages in cases that were identical except as to whether or not the error had been disclosed, those cases in which disclosure occurred resulted in much smaller judgments. In the context of disclosure, these mock juries apparently focused more on meeting the needs of the patient than on punishing the physician or hospital.[129]

As further evidence, several organizations that have adopted disclosure policies have reported a favorable financial impact from open disclosure policies. One widely cited example (discussed in more detail below) is that of the VA Medical Center in Lexington, Kentucky. Its data, which have received wide exposure, show that its open disclosure policy and proactive stance have not resulted in greater litigation costs than among its peers within the VA system that do not have these policies.[96,130–133] Some have suggested, however, that the Veterans Health Administration is not representative of the U.S. health care system overall, given that all of its health care practitioners are employed by the government and therefore not personally liable. However, these physicians can still be reported to the National Practitioner Data Bank and state systems, and many of these physicians practice in both University and VA hospitals, making the Lexington experience somewhat more generalizable.

Another institution well known for its disclosure policy is the University of Michigan. Richard Boothman, who became chief risk officer in 2001, brought to the university his belief, based on many years as a trial lawyer defending health care clients, that the process of handling patients' complaints and claims that often involved legal action could be much improved.[130,134] Initial efforts to reduce claims at the University of Michigan were undertaken—and then expanded to include an examination of how inadequate attention to patient safety and "unmindful patient communication" contributed to the malpractice "crisis." The university began to focus on what it considered primary causes for patient litigation, namely, "a failure to be accountable when warranted and a reluctance to communicate." Key principles were constructed and applied: the university would compensate patients quickly and fairly if injury was caused by inappropriate medical care; it would defend appropriate care; and it would use mistakes to learn and improve. Openness and transparency with patients (and their lawyers) were found to benefit all parties, leading to fair settlements and reducing litigation.

As described by Boothman, the university has had a disclosure policy since 2002. The approach has three components:

1. Acknowledge cases in which a patient was hurt because of medical error and compensate these patients quickly and fairly.
2. Aggressively defend cases that the hospital considers to be without merit.
3. Study all adverse events to determine how procedures could be improved.

A schematic flowchart of the university's process is shown in figure 3.

The financial impact of its program is impressive and was cited by Hilary Rodham Clinton and Barack Obama in an article they wrote on medical liability reform in the *New England Journal of Medicine* in 2006.[2] As shown in figure 4, annual litigation costs were cut from $3 million to $1 million, the average time to resolution of claims and lawsuits went from 20 months to 9 months, and the annual number of claims and lawsuits dropped from 262 to 114.[2,130]

But these reports from isolated hospitals and health care systems may not tell the whole story. Some regard it as common sense that if patients and families were told about errors that otherwise would have remained hidden, many of them would decide to sue. Furthermore, while many lawsuits are baseless, this new group of lawsuits would be brought as a result of the disclosure of the hospitals and the clinicians, therefore giving

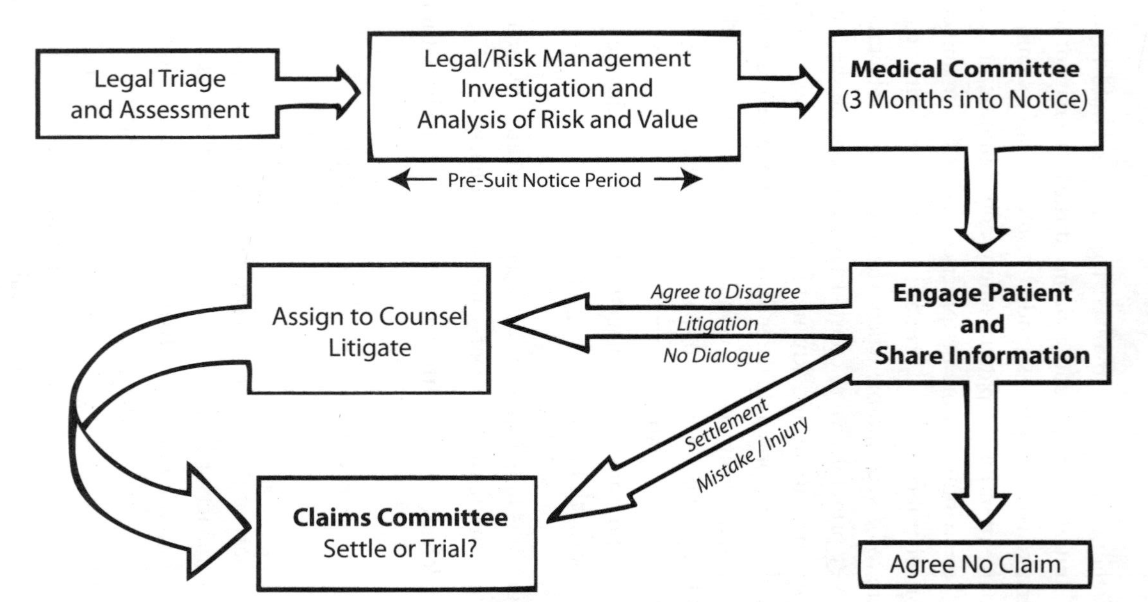

FIGURE 3. Claims management model at the University of Michigan. *Source:* Boothman R, Blackwell A, Campbell D, Commiskey E, Anderson S. A better approach to medical malpractice claims? The University of Michigan experience. *J Health Life Sciences Law.* 2009;2:125–159

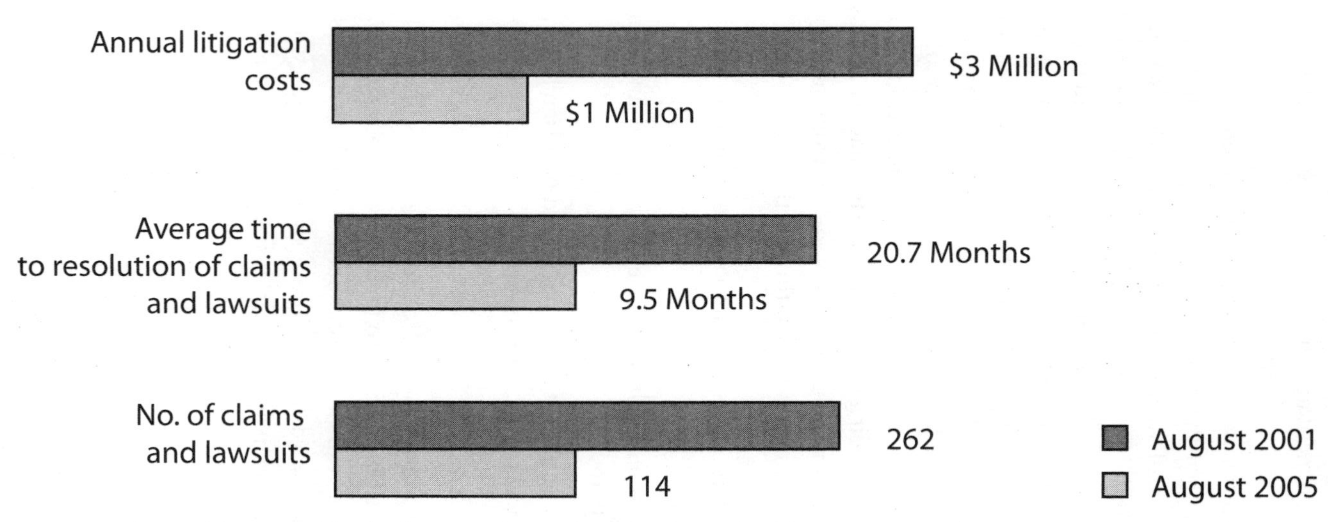

FIGURE 4. Financial impact of the disclosure policy at the University of Michigan. *Source:* Clinton HR, Obama B. Making patient safety the centerpiece of medical liability reform. *N Engl J Med.* 2006;354:2205–2208

them credibility and merit and making it likely that they would be expensive to resolve.

This is indeed the conclusion reached by Studdert and colleagues at the Harvard School of Public Health in their article entitled "Disclosure of Medical Injury to Patients: An Improbable Risk Management Strategy."[135] In this article they refer to "the great unlitigated reservoir," noting that "the number of serious injuries that do not lead to claims dwarfs the number that do." Furthermore, they observe that our medical malpractice system is sustained by the fact that while severe injuries are prevalent, most never trigger litigation. They therefore undertook an analysis using Monte Carlo simulation of large databases on medical injury drawn from New York, Utah, and Colorado. They examined a number of hypothetical scenarios, including the likelihood that proactive disclosure would diminish the size of the judgments as predicted from mock trial studies. Under optimistic conditions, they estimated that

- disclosure would more than double the number of claims and lawsuits;
- disclosure would reduce the size of awards by an average of 40 percent; and
- the overall impact of disclosure would be a significant, but modest, increase in compensation costs from $5.8 to 7.0 billion/year.

The Harvard researchers concluded their analysis by acknowledging that "disclosure is the right thing to do [and] so is compensating patients who sustain injury as a result of substandard care." Nonetheless, they note that "movement toward full disclosure should proceed with a realistic expectation of the financial implications and prudent planning to meet them."

Changes in Evidentiary Rules: The "Apology Laws"

As noted above, statements by a clinician may typically be introduced into evidence in a malpractice suit to help prove the plaintiff's case. As a result, clinicians may be reluctant to share information, express sympathy, or apologize based on a concern that their comments may be used against them. To remove or reduce this potential barrier to improving the response to injured patients, 35 states so far have passed laws that protect statements made by a practitioner from being used against the practitioner in court.[136,137] These so-called apology laws differ in the scope and content of what is protected. Some offer protection only for the statement of sympathy, while explicitly stating that admissions of fault are not protected. Other statutes also protect admissions of error or fault. For example, under the 2003 Colorado statute, which offers broad protection, if a patient brings an action in response to an unanticipated outcome of medical care, any statements, conduct, or gestures of the caregivers offering sympathy or making an apology for the death, injury, or suffering of the patient (made to the patient or the patient's family) cannot be introduced into evidence as an admission of liability.

The apology laws have been criticized for, among other things, (1) being insufficient to provide adequate protection, (2) singling out one group of professionals as needing protection from their own honest statements, (3) making it harder for patients to prove in court what their caregivers have already admitted, and (4) fostering insincere, strategic apologies.[116,125,136,137] Even the broadest apology law does not mean that the disclosure process might not lead to a lawsuit, especially if the disclosure and apology are what bring the error to the patient's attention. Some commentators urge that communications with patients be guided by ethical standards regardless of the existence (or not) of broad apology laws. Some of the most successful disclosure and apology programs have taken root at institutions located in states without apology laws, such as the University of Michigan (see fig. 4).[130] Nonetheless, these laws may provide comfort to some clinicians who are reluctant to disclose because of concern that their words will be used in court against them. More discussion of the role of apology in communicating about adverse events can be found in the sections below.

The Development of Programs and Policies

Numerous institutions have responded to the call for greater disclosure of information about adverse events. Eve Shapiro prepared a summary of several of these programs for a Robert Wood Johnson Foundation–supported workshop in 2006. A summary of her research into programs at the Lexington, Kentucky, Veterans Administration, the University of Michigan, Kaiser Permanente, Geisinger Health System, Catholic Health Initiatives, and COPIC Insurance Company is provided below,[138] with additional information in table 4.[139]

The program at the VA Medical Center in Lexington, Kentucky, discussed above, had its origin in two malpractice cases in 1987 that resulted in significant monetary damages. In response, the center developed a policy of open communication regarding adverse events. In 1995, the Department of Veterans Affairs adopted a general policy of informing patients of adverse events and providing assurances about what steps would be taken to minimize further harm to the patient.[140] In March 2003, the National Ethics Committee for the VA system issued a report entitled "Disclosing Adverse Events to Patients," which summarized the ethical and legal rationale for disclosure, clarified what constitutes an adverse event, and described in more detail what needs to be disclosed, by whom, and when.

As of 2008, the VA continues to have a policy of disclosing adverse events to patients, including events that may not be obvious and events in which harm has not yet manifested itself but may do so in the future (disclosure of "near misses" is not mandated but depends on the situation). Their approach features categories of disclosure. The first is called "clinical disclosure," which consists of sharing clinical information with patients and families, expressing empathy, and assuring that an investigation will be conducted and steps taken to prevent similar occurrences in the future. Clinical disclosure is to be considered a routine part of care following an adverse event. Another category is "institutional disclosure," which occurs when an adverse event has resulted in serious harm or death or involves potential legal liability. Institutional disclosure is a more formal process that may include an apology and information about compensation for the patient's harm.[141]

In response to the IOM report *To Err Is Human,* Kaiser Permanente, which accepted the ethical obligation of communicating openly and honestly with patients after adverse events, took additional steps to carry out this commitment. Kaiser developed a detailed policy statement for

TABLE 4. Developments in Programs and Policies

Veterans Health Administration	Lexington, Kentucky, VA adopted policy of "extreme honesty" in 1987, disclosure policy disseminated throughout the VA system in 2003
University of Michigan	Open disclosure since 2002. Three components: compensate patients quickly and fairly, aggressively defend cases that the hospital considers to be without merit, study all adverse events to determine how procedures could be improved
COPIC Insurance Company in Colorado	In 2000 adopted the "3Rs" program, involves "recognizing" an unanticipated event, "responding promptly," and "resolving" related issues. COPIC trains and supports physicians in communicating openly with patients, and financial assistance is available to patients on a "no fault" basis
Kaiser Permanente	Created "situation management teams" to help clinicians respond to adverse events, trained physicians in disclosure skills, offered peer support for clinicians, created the position of health care ombudsman to serve as the link between the clinicians and the patient/family
Geisinger Health System	A "core team" is available to help clinicians have open communications with their patients following adverse events. Virtually all physicians go through some kind of training for disclosing adverse events
Brigham and Women's Hospital in Boston	Recently created a comprehensive administrative structure, the Center for Professionalism and Peer Support, to provide disclosure coaching and peer support to clinicians
University of Illinois Medical Center at Chicago	Adopted Michigan-style disclosure program in 2006. A "Patient Communication Consult Service" assists clinicians with disclosure, and a "Care for the Care Giver" program provides peer support
Stanford University	Launched "Process for the Early Assessment and Resolution of Loss" (PEARL) in 2007, including a process to provide early compensation
Harvard Medical School–CRICO/RMF	Developed and disseminated "When Things Go Wrong" disclosure policy in 2006 and has offered training to more than 400 disclosure "coaches" throughout the Harvard system

Sources: Shapiro E. Disclosing medical errors: best practices from the "leading edge." March 2008. www.ihi.org/IHI/Topics/PatientSafety/SafetyGeneral/Literature. Accessed January 22, 2009. Gallagher TH. A 62-year-old woman with skin cancer who experienced wrong-site surgery: review of medical error. *JAMA*. 2009;302:669–677.

physicians about what to do after an adverse event. It also created "situation management teams" to help clinicians respond to adverse events and trained individual physicians in communication skills. Kaiser offered peer support for clinicians and created the position of health care ombudsman (a certified health care mediator, who serves as the link between the health care team and the patient/family).

Geisinger Health System's disclosure policy was initially prompted by a new legal requirement that a person who was injured or died as a result of medical negligence have a prompt review of the case and fair compensation and that patient injuries be reduced by identifying problems and implementing solutions. After passage of the law, Geisinger implemented a policy of communicating errors and adverse outcomes to patients. This policy became more than a response to a legal requirement and soon evolved into a commitment to involve patients more fully in all aspects of their care. A "core team" was trained to participate in and help clinicians have open communications with their patients following adverse events. Geisinger reports that over time virtually all its physicians go through some kind of training for disclosing adverse events.

Reflecting a long-held value of compassionate communication, Catholic Health Initiatives (CHI) adopted a model disclosure policy in 2006. The ethical bases for the policy include the desires and moral claims of patients and families and the imperative to improve patient care and safety. While the policy itself need not be adopted by every hospital in the CHI system, it does advocate compassion and encourage apology throughout the system. Fair compensation for harm caused by error is a part of the process. Although the policy was adopted primarily to reflect core values, the disclosure approach also appears to have helped reduce losses related to adverse events.

Brigham and Women's Hospital in Boston adopted its policy of routinely disclosing adverse events and errors in 2002. Recently it has created a comprehensive administrative structure to support this process, the Center for Professionalism and Peer Support, under the direction of Dr. Jo Shapiro, the chief of the Division of Otolaryngology. There are four initiatives within the center. One is focused on education about professionalism, with mandatory workshops covering topics like sexual misconduct and disruptive behavior. Another is focused on disclosure coaching. In addition to recruiting and providing ongoing education for a cohort of institutional coaches, this initiative also conducts a number of educational programs, such as grand rounds, to make the hospital community aware of the hospital's commitment to open disclosure and the availability of the coaches as essential resources. Third, the center provides peer-support services, both as a routine mechanism for following up with clinicians who are involved in an error or other potentially traumatic event, and in assisting those who need more intensive support and professional services. Finally, the center has a "defendant support program," whereby the hospital leadership reaches out to those who have been named in a lawsuit to reassure them that the institution will stand with them throughout the process and to mitigate any sense the clinicians may have that they could be ostracized by the legal allegations.[142]

In 2000, COPIC Insurance Company, which insures physicians in Colorado, adopted a voluntary early intervention program. The "3Rs" program, applicable to cases that do not involve death or clear negligence, involves "recognizing" an unanticipated event, "responding promptly," and "resolving" related issues. Physicians are encouraged to report cases immediately and to begin the 3Rs process. To facilitate this process, COPIC trains and supports physicians in communicating openly with patients and providing patients with information and emotional support. Financial assistance is available to patients for health care expenses and loss of time, on a "no fault" basis. Patients are also told what will be done to prevent a recurrence of the adverse event. When appropriate, an apology is offered. About half of the insured physicians participate, and this group has experienced no greater claims than the other half, and perhaps fewer. Patient and physician satisfaction is high, and outcomes appear to show that adverse events handled through this program are resolved more amicably than if they were litigated. Further, the payments in each case have been relatively modest.[96,143] Key elements of the COPIC program are shown in table 5.

In interpreting the data from the University of Michigan and other programs that offer compensation as a part of their risk management strategy, it is difficult or impossible to tease out how much of the success is related to the practice of open disclosure and how much might be related to their proactive approach of offering early compensation. In fact, there is some evidence to suggest that the disclosure process is not primarily responsible for driving any increase in satisfaction.

TABLE 5. The COPIC 3Rs Program

Key Features
Disclosure linked to no-fault compensation for patient's out-of-pocket expenses (up to $30,000)
Disclosure training for physicians
Exclusion criteria: death, clear negligence, attorney involvement, complaint to state board, written demand for payment
Disclosure coaching for physician and case management for patient provided by 3Rs administrators
Payments not reportable to National Practitioner Data Bank
Key Outcomes (January 2000–October 2006)
2,853 Colorado physicians enrolled
3,200 events handled in program
25% of patients received payments; average, $5,400 per case
Seven paid cases subsequently litigated, two of which resulted in tort compensation
16 unpaid cases subsequently litigated, 6 of which resulted in tort compensation

Source: Gallagher TH, Studdert D, Levinson W. Disclosing harmful medical errors to patients. *N Engl J Med.* 2007;356:2713–2719.

These are just a few examples of the movement toward full disclosure in health care organizations. As early as 2004, it was estimated that "most" hospitals had a written policy for informing patients or families of a preventable medical error.[55,144] Eighty-one percent of respondents in one study reported either the existence of an error disclosure policy at their hospital or one in the making.[145] It can be argued that even in the absence of a legal mandate to disclose, the existence of such a policy is likely to become the "standard" in the industry.

While the adoption of policies is promising, for such policies to result in a substantial change in disclosure practice they must be accompanied by a change in the organizational culture itself. This change requires not only dissemination of the hospital's policy of transparency but also the creation of a nonpunitive environment for disclosure, the development of training and support for clinicians, support for patients and families, and the "buy in" of all the stakeholders within the system.[6,42]

FIVE

Supporting Clinicians in Disclosure

The Coaching Model

The increasing emphasis on the importance of disclosure over the past few years has led many organizations to undertake programs to develop policies and procedures, as well as to begin educating their health care workers about this issue. At Harvard, the emphasis on disclosure was renewed in 2006 when Harvard Medical School produced the highly influential consensus document *When Things Go Wrong* under the leadership of Lucian L. Leape, a pediatric surgeon and nationally respected leader in the patient safety movement.[6] This document, endorsed by all the Harvard teaching hospitals, promotes a policy of openness, fairness, and honesty in communicating with patients and families about adverse events and medical errors.

Having a policy is, of course, an important first step. Yet documents and policies alone do not create an effective practice. Furthermore, disclosure conversations are significantly more complex and difficult than almost any other conversation that occurs in health care. Telling people they have just suffered a stroke is hard enough, but having to tell them that the stroke was caused by a mistake, for which you or your colleagues are responsible, is substantially more difficult. Deciding how to share the facts of the situation and avoid speculation while simultaneously managing feelings of guilt, the urge to assign blame, and the desire to protect oneself is hardly an easy task.

Dr. Leape was one of the first to recognize these challenges associated with translating the Harvard policy into practice. He had the vision to promote the development of an educational curriculum, based on concepts in adult learning, to develop a cohort of clinicians who were highly competent in the knowledge and relational competencies necessary to skillfully engage patients and families in these conversations.

As a result of his insight and efforts, the Institute for Professionalism and Ethical Practice at Children's Hospital Boston and Harvard's CRICO/RMF formed a partnership to address the question: What is the most pragmatic approach to teaching clinicians how to effectively and skillfully engage with patients and families in these conversations? Similar efforts were under way at other institutions, stemming from Dr. Gallagher and colleagues' research and teaching program on disclosure that began at Washington University in St. Louis and continues at the University of Washington.

The development of the curriculum followed a sequential process. First, we identified the range of skills necessary to effectively improve practice in this area of medicine. In addition to the capacity for empathy and emotional connection, clinicians need to have a firm understanding of their hospital's policies and disclosure standards. They need to recognize the powerful impact of medical error on themselves and the other clinicians involved and be able to identify those situations in which a colleague may need to be removed from the clinical situation for the sake of the patient as well as for their own well-being. They need to be aware of and be prepared to handle the range of emotions that the patient and family may experience and project, such as fear, anger, and denial. Finally, they need to be familiar with the various resources and support services available at the hospital and how to access them.

Another dilemma was created by the fact that all the Harvard hospitals have hundreds, even thousands, of clinicians who at any time could become involved in a serious medical error. On the one hand, any effective educational strategy must involve a broad-based learning initiative designed to provide all these clinicians with a general understanding of the hospital's approach to disclosure, particularly in view of the fact that most of these clinicians were trained to withhold any information from patients that might convey wrongdoing or liability. On the other hand, we realized that it would be unrealistic to think that any educational program could enable this huge number of clinicians to learn and retain the knowledge needed to have these conversations well at any moment in time. Therefore we decided to endorse an approach that would assure the "just-in-time" availability of expertise and help by concentrating our

TABLE 6. Key Elements of the Safe Practice Guideline on Disclosure from the National Quality Forum

Content to Be Disclosed to the Patient
Provide facts about the event
Presence of error or system failure, if known
Results of event analysis to support informed decision making by the patient
Express regret for unanticipated outcome
Give formal apology if unanticipated outcome is caused by error or system failure
Institutional Requirements
Integrate disclosure, patient safety, and risk management activities
Establish disclosure support system
Provide background disclosure education
Ensure that disclosure coaching is available at all times
Provide emotional support for health care workers, administrators, patients, and families
Use performance-improvement tools to track and enhance disclosure

Source: Gallagher TH, Studdert D, Levinson W. Disclosing harmful medical errors to patients. *N Engl J Med.* 2007;356:2713–2719.

educational efforts on a small number of disclosure "coaches" who would be available to all clinicians within the institution on a 24/7 basis.

Simultaneous with our struggle regarding the development of an educational strategy, the National Quality Forum (NQF) promulgated a "safe practice guideline" for disclosure that incorporated many of the same elements that we adopted (table 6).[95] Specifically, one key aspect of the NQF model is the availability of disclosure coaches at all times. The model envisions these coaches to be respected individuals throughout the institution, known for their negotiation and people skills, who would have the training and experience necessary to provide their clinician colleagues with competent, high-quality advice and education on a just-in-time basis.

Organizing Support for Disclosure within Institutions

Beyond the general skills and characteristics required for a disclosure coach, one important and still largely unanswered question relates to the types of clinicians most appropriate for this role. Current practice seems to be highly variable. We are aware of one community hospital in which the hospital president insists on being involved in all adverse events and disclosure conversations. In some hospitals, professional risk managers (often with a background in nursing) already seem to be functioning extremely well with many of the skill sets that we have identified as essential for the coaching role. At other hospitals, however, risk managers are recognized more for their expertise in the analysis of adverse events and in making complex but technical recommendations regarding potential liability, reportability, and the like rather than for their ability to help clinicians have these difficult conversations.

Based on our understanding of the literature and our experience in the field, we offer two general recommendations:

1. The personal characteristics, skills, and knowledge of the individuals chosen to be coaches are more important than their specific roles or titles within the institution. Regardless of whether they are risk managers, hospital presidents, nursing leaders, or division chiefs, their most important attributes are the degree to which they are trusted, available, and capable of providing high-quality counseling and advice to their colleagues.
2. All individuals who function in the coaching role must recognize that they do not function independently but must integrate seamlessly into the hospital's risk management structure, the institution's programs on quality and safety, and the relationship between the hospital, clinicians, and their malpractice carriers. The coach must enjoy enough stature and independence within the institution so that his or her recommendations are not overly influenced by the drive to minimize liability but must also appreciate that operating entirely outside the hospital's risk management program and guidelines would be reckless. Excellent disclosure programs should ensure a close working relationship between the hospital coaches and the risk management department.

Another question that has not yet been fully resolved is what the best model will be for providing coaching expertise across health care organizations. We have seen two emerging options that integrate and build on existing consultation models within hospitals that so far hold the most promise:

1. Over the past several decades, ethics consultation services in hospitals throughout the United States have largely evolved from being seen as threatening intrusions into the authority of attending physicians to being a welcomed and well-regarded source of help and expertise for troubling cases. Disclosure coaching and ethics consultation share a number of features—both rely on a discrete area of expertise as well as the need for excellent judgment and discretion. Therefore, some institutions have chosen to frame their disclosure support in terms of a "communication consult service" and have structured these services using methods of access and documentation parallel to ethics consultation.
2. More recently, many hospitals have developed "rapid response teams" for emergent events that occur within the hospital, primarily when patients suffer acute clinical deterioration. An important part of the philosophy behind these teams is that, regardless of the expertise of the clinicians already involved in the care of the patient, the management of these crises can always be improved with help from "extra hands" who bring an outside perspective and additional skills. Some institutions have therefore chosen to frame their disclosure programs on the model of crisis response—for example, by promoting activation of an on-call beeper system when clinicians are faced with a disclosure "emergency."

At this point, our view is that the best model has yet to be well defined and that individual institutions should begin with an approach that best fits with their existing culture and resources and then make modifications over time based on the usefulness and performance of the approach.

Whatever approach is taken, however, a common principle is that patients and families want to have the primary conversations with their clinicians, not with coaches, risk managers, or other institutional representatives. The primary role of the coach is to assist these clinicians in how to have this conversation well, not to insert themselves directly into the disclosure process. While coaches may, at times, determine that one or more of the clinicians involved is not capable of having a skillful and appropriate conversation with the patient or family, in general the job of the coach is to facilitate the abilities of the clinicians to engage in these conversations, not to displace them.

An Educational Curriculum for Disclosure Coaches

The workshops that we have designed and taught are consistent with the NQF coaching model. We focus especially on understanding and practicing the coaching role through the lens of leadership and the lens of learning. To effect change in health care organizations vis-à-vis how patients and families are engaged in the aftermath of adverse events, the coach must be an effective leader, with the personal authority and relational competence that successful leaders must have. As an institutional leader who is trying to advance a new practice, the coach is also a key facilitator of learning, a hands-on clinical educator who promotes the values, knowledge, and skillfulness that physicians and other health care professionals must engage in throughout the organization in order to develop and implement this evolving practice of disclosure.

As an institutional leader and facilitator of learning, the coach holds a vision of positive organizational change with respect to how mistakes and failures should be handled, implicitly and explicitly challenging a medical culture in which historically mistakes have been seen as purely negative events that should be kept secret. In this respect, the coach is a proponent of a new attitude within medical culture toward error, one based on a new appreciation for the "aesthetic of imperfection" as a critical pathway toward safety in health care organizations.[146] When an adverse event occurs, a skillful coach needs to step into the situation with not only an understanding of how things are but also an appreciation for how they might become. Skillful coaches need to be cognizant that their own behavior—the degree of transparency, respect, accountability, continuity, and kindness they bring to the process—will role-model the attributes they are hoping will be enacted in the disclosure conversation with the patient and family.[147] Like other artful forms of teaching in clinical medical education, this is a learning intervention occurring in real time, focusing on real practice. The clinicians who engage in this kind of relational learning receive a powerful message of how things are changing with regard to transparency with patients and families, and they are invited and empowered, in the context of a compelling clinical situation, to be part of that change.

When a significant adverse event occurs, the coach is by definition intervening in a clinical situation in which the moral and emotional stakes are high for clinicians, patients, and family members alike. Thus there is a high likelihood for a potent learning experience, one that will be either growth-promoting or growth-hindering for the clinicians involved. At a time historically when medical institutions are in enormous flux in terms of how they go about addressing adverse events and medical errors, a skillful coaching intervention can result in powerful learning that is likely to stick with the involved clinicians in an unparalleled way, due to the moral and emotional salience of the event. Also, because it is literally a "critical incident" in the process of unfolding, this real-time intervention provides a potentially powerful initial step in a learning process that will evolve over time and incorporate retroactive reflection in the days and weeks to come.[148]

SIX

Practice-Based Learning for Coaches and Clinicians

In designing an educational curriculum for disclosure, our task was to craft learning activities that would incorporate the values, skills, and knowledge relevant both to having conversations with patients and families in the aftermath of adverse events and medical errors and to helping clinicians prepare for such conversations. In this section, we describe what we have been teaching and what we have learned so far. The relational and practice-based approach we bring to our educational activities was developed through many years of experience designing and conducting educational workshops focused on difficult conversations in health care.[149,150] We also situate our educational approach in a body of recent scholarship focused on how to understand and cultivate optimal organizational learning in health care settings.[151–153]

Aristotle differentiated between *phronesis,* or skillfulness in practice, and *episteme,* or theoretical knowledge. Theoretical knowledge is important, but it is empty unless linked to practical knowledge. This principle is applicable throughout medicine: for example, theoretical knowledge of anatomy and pathophysiology is necessary to become a competent surgeon but is valueless unless coupled with the practical understanding that develops over years of managing real cases. Striking the right balance between phronesis and episteme has been especially important in the design and implementation of our educational activities because the capacities we want to strengthen—conveying kindness, thinking clearly, and communicating well in situations fraught with conflict and emotion—emerge largely from the personal and professional "experience banks" of seasoned clinicians. Competence, in this context, is less about mastering a toolkit full of behavioral skills and more about developing a flexible capacity to enact key values and knowledge in always new and changing situations.

Therefore, a key component of our approach is to emphasize the idea that the activities of disclosure and coaching are not brand new; rather, they are built on various practices, largely informal and generally unexamined, already in existence. Department chiefs, nursing supervisors, and others have developed a range of ways of responding to adverse events, including the provision of guidance to clinicians most centrally involved. We see our workshops as an opportunity to place these practices in front of us, in a safe and respectful learning environment, so that we can, first, learn what may already be working well and second, reflect together on how the practice can be improved.

Becoming adept in these new practices of disclosure and coaching is analogous, in many ways, to the process by which clinicians gain proficiency in managing ethical dilemmas. While a theoretical understanding of ethical principles and theories is invaluable to clinical ethicists in their training, competence in this realm resides in real-world practice with actual cases. Virtually all clinical ethics programs, therefore, build learning activities around the discussion of particular cases, using the details and contextual features of each case as the primary scaffold for exploring the relevant ethical considerations.

How should clinicians go about learning these new communication practices? First, they need to explore the core relational values that will inform the practices—values that build (and rebuild) health care relationships. Second, they need to know how to act with kindness, by providing a compassionate and empathic response to others that is sensitive to the emotional impact of these events. Third, they need to appreciate the role and importance of apology. Fourth, they need to know how to approach these conversations as collaborative and interactive events. Fifth, they need to know how to discern and balance the perspectives of patients, families, and clinicians, as well as to understand the organizational culture that surrounds them. Sixth, they need practical guidelines to assist and support them in the new practice. Last, they need a safe, respectful learning setting in which to enact these new practices in the company of peers.

We begin with an ethical mandate. While ethical arguments do not by themselves necessarily change behavior, we believe it is important to reach clinicians as both human beings *and* professionals. Therefore, we start our educational work with the message that the first reason we need to do a better job of responding to patients, families and clinicians in the aftermath of adverse events and medical errors is because—as Lucian Leape has argued for many years—it is the right thing to do.

Medical errors involve a series of events occurring within a network of human relationships that are themselves guided and informed by values. What are the values at the core of these relationships? How can these values be enacted to *rebuild* relationships in the aftermath of a medical error? We have identified five core relational values—transparency, respect, accountability, continuity, and kindness—that are referred to by the acronym TRACK (table 7). We believe these values, when enacted robustly, can serve as an ethical roadmap for clinicians to help them "track" the process of rebuilding relationships that have been disrupted or ruptured by the occurrence of a medical error. These values are relevant to the needs of *all* individuals impacted by the event—whether patient, family member, or clinician.

In line with calls from many quarters within health care, we first emphasize the overarching value of transparency.[1,154,155] Many commentators argue that increased transparency, in the form of greater access to any relevant information affecting patients' health, is fundamental to the changes the health care system must undergo if it is to maintain the trust of patients and families in the twenty-first century.

Donald Berwick, a prominent national leader in health care quality improvement, describes the value of transparency as follows: "I cannot imagine a future health care system in which we do not work in daylight, study openly what we do, and offer patients any windows they want onto the work that affects them. 'No secrets' is the new rule."[154] In the aftermath of an adverse event or medical error, working in daylight with patients and families takes on vital importance. One of the first needs for patients and families at these times is to be able to understand and make sense of what has happened. It is the responsibility of clinicians to help

TABLE 7. The TRACK Acronym

Core Relational Value	Definition	Optimal Practical Outcome
Transparency	The quality of being open, frank, obvious	I've had timely access to the information and input I've needed.
Respect	Esteem for the worth or excellence of a person	I've been valued as a human being by the people helping me.
Accountability	The state of being answerable or called to account	The right people have assumed responsibility for their actions.
Continuity	The property of a continuous and connected period of time	The care I've received makes sense and fits together.
Kindness	The quality of acting with caring and consideration	I've been treated with warmth, empathy, and compassion.

Source: Copyright 2007 Institute for Professionalism and Ethical Practice and Harvard Risk Management Foundation.

them with this task, even in situations in which all the facts are not yet known, and continue to provide an open flow of relevant information in the days and weeks that follow.

Table 7 provides simple definitions for the five core values, as well as an optimal practical outcome for each. We invite coaches and clinicians to envision how, in the aftermath of an adverse event, we might know whether each value has been successfully enacted. In other words, what would be an ideal outcome in practice?

If we were to check in with a clinician, patient, or family member impacted by the event, at any point in the weeks and months that follow, and we were to inquire about the degree of frankness and openness experienced by that person in the process, we might expect to hear in response: "I've had timely access to the information and input I've needed." In terms of respect, we might hope to learn: "I've been valued as a human being by the people helping me." If the individuals responding to the event were answerable and accountable in appropriate ways, we might anticipate being told: "The right people have assumed responsibility for their actions." If the process of interaction was continuous and coherent, we might expect to be informed: "The care I've received makes sense and fits together." Last, if we were to inquire about kindness, we might hope to hear: "I've been treated with warmth and caring."

Acting with Kindness: Compassion and Empathy

> Kindness is compassion in action. It is a way of taking the vital human emotions of empathy or sympathy and channeling those emotions into a real-life confrontation with ruthlessness, abandonment, thoughtlessness, loneliness—all the myriad ways, every single day, we find ourselves suffering or witnessing suffering in others.
>
> SHARON SALZBERG, *The Force of Kindness: Change Your Life with Love and Compassion*

We stress the importance of kindness as a core relational value that captures the fundamental importance of being willing to see, acknowledge, and bear witness to the suffering of patients, family members, and clinicians who have been part of an adverse event or medical error. Especially when the event is serious and significant harm has been done, it is critical to engage with patients, family members, and clinicians not only on a cognitive level, helping them to make sense of what has happened, but also on an emotional level, helping them to absorb and express the emotional impact of the event. We have found that the most difficult question for clinicians to ask family members in the aftermath of these events are is "How is this for you?" or "What is hardest about this for you?" Perhaps the difficulty with asking the question is connected to the difficulty in hearing the answer, which is likely to be one that conveys fear, sadness, and anger, not to mention acute disappointment in the clinician or health care team.

Acting with kindness can take the form of compassion, which means, literally, "to suffer with." While none of us can presume to understand fully the experience of another person who is suffering, we can connect to that person from the place within us that knows suffering in our own lives. Acting with kindness can also take the form of empathy, which is more an effort to actively imagine what another person is experiencing by trying to put oneself into the head and heart of that person in the hope of understanding what he or she, uniquely, is going through.

In the medical world, empathy is sometimes taught as a technique or a rehearsed behavior one shows to patients and families as opposed to a genuine effort to understand and, through understanding, to be moved by their suffering. We have found that patients and family members, especially those who have just experienced a traumatic medical event, are rather adept at knowing the difference. This is not to say that it is wrong to teach communication skills that can be helpful in health care encounters, only that it is the humanness underlying those skills that ultimately will matter.

Collaborative Conversations

The immediate aftermath of a medical error is often a time fraught with high emotions on the part of patients, family members, and clinicians alike. Strong emotions can distort clinicians' judgment about whether an adverse event took place, whether that adverse event was due to an error, and if so how this information should be shared with the patient and family. These factors lead to interactive exchanges—whether the conversations between a coach and team of clinicians or the conversations among clinicians, the patient, and family members—that are inherently challenging. The particular way in which a coach communicates with clinicians in the aftermath of an event will sets a powerful tone and precedent for the way in which the clinicians will then approach the patient and family.

The temptation in these conversations, given that the stakes are so high, is for coaches to behave too much like traditional experts, acting under the assumption that they need to quickly transfer large chunks of information and guidance to clinicians so they will quickly absorb what they need to know and do. Clinicians face an analogous temptation when they speak with the patient and family, often focusing too exclusively on delivering information without appreciating sufficiently the broader human event that is under way.

While conveying information coherently is indeed a central aspect of coaching as well as the process of communicating with the patient and family, succeeding at this task depends on developing a broader appreciation of the *kind* of conversation that needs to take place. The word "conversation" is derived from the Latin *conversari*, which means to keep company, dwell in a place, or live with. From our standpoint as educators, we want coaches to *keep company* with clinicians when these events take place. We want clinicians to *dwell* in the place patients and families inhabit when they are told about a medical error. And we want coaches and clinicians alike to *live with* the complex and very real human drama that unfolds in the aftermath of a serious event. To be successful, the conversation that coaches have with clinicians or that clinicians have with patients and families must be a *collaborative* one. Its outcome should not be under the control or ownership of any one contributor; rather, it needs to "belong" to *all* participants.

One useful tool for helping coaches and clinicians stay connected to the interactive and collaborative nature of these conversations is the ask-tell-ask method.[156] This approach involves *asking* individuals what they understand about a particular situation, *telling* them additional, targeted information in a way that incorporates their current understanding and is comprehensible, and then *asking* how they understand and feel about the information that has been offered. When coaches are talking with clinicians who have been part of an event, or when clinicians are talking with patients and family members who are involved, less is very often more, in that what needs to be said should be shaped by the particular context, the information needed at particular moments in time, and the level of understanding that particular individuals bring to the conversation. When coaches are talking with clinicians in preparation for a conversation with a patient or family, they can explicitly review the ask-tell-ask approach, provide a concrete example of how the approach is used, and, if appropriate, invite clinicians to role-play the use of the approach in preparation for talking with the patient or family. Putting the ask-tell-ask method into practice can help coaches and clinicians concentrate on the "back-and-forthness" of successful conversations and avoid the temptation to talk too much and listen too little.[156]

Caring and Apology

The recent literature on disclosure is replete with the recommendation that clinicians should apologize and say "I'm sorry" to patients and families when there has been an adverse event.[127,133,157–160] We believe there has been confusion in professional discourse about disclosure that results from the tendency to equate two different kinds of communication: saying "I'm sorry" as an expression of caring and saying "I'm sorry" as an apology for one's own actions or the actions of one's organization.[116,139,161]

We agree wholeheartedly that the words "I'm sorry" (as in "I'm so sorry this happened"), conveyed authentically, can be a crucial part of an empathic and compassionate response to patients and family members who have gone through a traumatic medical event. These words, which have been used throughout human history when something bad happens to someone one cares about, are quite important for patients and families to hear following an adverse event, regardless of whether there has been a medical error. Sadly, the words "I'm sorry" have in effect been stolen from clinicians as the result of decades of advice from attorneys and risk managers, the essence of which has been: whatever else you do in these situations, make sure to never say you're sorry. We encourage coaches and clinicians to reclaim these words, along with the requisite human genuineness that give the words moral salience and meaning.

At the same time, we emphasize a second learning point. Saying "I'm sorry" as an expression of caring after a serious unhoped-for medical outcome that is not the result of medical error is a different communication, with a different meaning, than saying "I'm sorry" when a clinician needs to take responsibility for individual or organizational actions, small or large, that could have been avoided or should have been better than they were.[162] For this reason, we think it is helpful to restrict use of the term "apology" for these latter situations involving clinical or organizational accountability. At these times, an apology (as in "I'm so sorry this happened—I/we made a mistake for which I/we are responsible" or "This was an error on my/our part, and I want to apologize to you") is critically important.[162] Of course, the gravity of the apology and degree of sincere regret or remorse expressed should be commensurate with the severity of harm or potential harm.

We have found that distinguishing between these two kinds of communication can be freeing for coaches and clinicians because, first, it enables them to reclaim their natural capacity for caring and kindness in these interactions. Second, it focuses appropriate attention on the crucial importance of apologizing to patients and families when clinicians and the health care organizations of which they are a part need to assume accountability, whether for lesser incidents in which harm is negligible or for larger incidents in which the harm has been substantial. By stressing this distinction in the context of our core relational values, acting with kindness and apologizing each assume their rightful place, contextually, as key components of disclosure conversations.

Multiple Perspectives and Competing Ethics

Coaches and clinicians who become skillful at the practice of transparency are adept at seeing and understanding the perspectives of others.[163–165] Coaching clinicians in the aftermath of an event and communicating with patients and families at these times require the capacity to be knowledgeable about multiple perspectives as well as the ability to engage with multiple perspectives at the same time.

We believe three perspectives are particularly important to understand and appreciate: the perspective of patients and family members, the perspective of fellow clinicians, and the perspective of the organizational culture, which includes existing disclosure policies, administrative priorities in relation to transparency, risk management issues, and the overall tone and atmosphere of the organization vis-à-vis adverse events and medical errors. It is important to explore frankly how these diverse perspectives can be either in harmony or in conflict at various points in time.

Intervening effectively in the aftermath of an adverse event or medical error, especially in complex health care organizations, necessarily entails stepping into a range of competing ethics. Learning how to recognize, weigh, and balance these competing ethics is an important part of skillful practice. One example of competing ethics is the need for the patient and family to have a timely, plausible, and coherent explanation for what has happened as soon as possible versus the importance of clinicians avoiding speculation, steering clear of premature explanations, and carefully establishing "the facts" of what happened. Another instance of competing ethics emerges when a coach wants to have a physician in training who has been involved in an event take part in the disclosure conversation as part of his or her professional development but has to weigh that need with the question of whether the physician is in the proper emotional state to interact effectively with the patient and family. Keeping in mind the overriding rule, which is that the needs of the patient and family must come first, coaches and clinicians can weigh and strive to balance the competing ethics routinely embedded in these situations, thereby providing valuable mentorship for the clinical team as they strive to improve practice.

When asking clinicians to hold multiple perspectives and balance competing ethics, it is important to directly acknowledge the ways in which this invitation to new practice is embedded in change processes and priorities currently in motion within their health care organizations including, at times, barriers and obstacles that may have not yet been addressed. Each of the organizations we have worked with has developed new policies that support transparency in regard to adverse events and medical errors, but necessary reforms such as early compensation for patients and families and appropriate legal protection for clinicians who adopt a policy of full disclosure are, for the most part, not yet in place. It is important to acknowledge to clinicians that these issues are real and that addressing them will be a necessary part of the overall change process in order for the value of transparency to be fully actualized in health care organizations.

SEVEN

Practical Guidelines for Disclosure

In developing practical guidelines to assist and support coaches and clinicians, we began by reviewing and incorporating the information already available in the literature. Not surprisingly, a review of the ethics literature, empirical studies, and institutional policies suggests that while certain differences in approach exist, there is fairly widespread agreement about the elements that characterize good communication with patients and families that is likely to help preserve the patient-physician relationship and that may, at least in some cases, reduce the chance of legal action.

For example, Gallagher notes that the following represents the minimal information that should be conveyed after an error has occurred: (1) an explicit statement that an error occurred; (2) a basic description of what the error was, why the error happened, and how recurrences will be prevented; and (3) an apology.[15,21] The consensus statement adopted by the Harvard teaching hospitals, in addressing the "who, what, and when" of disclosure, recommends the following components of the communication: (1) telling the patient and family what happened, (2) taking responsibility, (3) expressing regret and apologizing when there has been an error, and (4) explaining what will be done to prevent similar events in the future.[6]

The National Quality Forum (NQF) has developed a similar list of elements that should be a part of a conversation with a patient after an adverse event. In addition to the steps outlined above, the NQF recommends timeliness of communication; follow-up with the results of any investigation; emotional support of patients, families, and clinicians; and education and skill building associated with creating a program of systems improvement, with special emphasis on building a just culture.[166]

Our guidelines for coaches and clinicians are also the product of our educational experience with health care professionals over several years. As a result of the ongoing dialogue between what we have taught and what we have learned, the guidelines have undergone a process of continual development and refinement. They are designed to be used as a "just-in-time" checklist. Many of the suggestions presume that someone has taken charge of the process and is able to provide guidance to the rest of the team. Ideally, this should be someone in a coaching role, but in hospitals that have not adopted this approach as an institutional model, it could be the attending or someone else in a position of clinical leadership. We refer to this person as the "coach," recognizing that this role may be filled in a variety of ways. An abbreviated version of the guidelines is included in the appendix, but here we explore them in detail.

First Priorities

- *Ensure that the clinical team stays fully attentive to the medical needs of the patient.*

  In the immediate aftermath of an adverse event, clinicians may not be sufficiently focused on the patient's medical needs, either because they are fearful of the patient's reaction or preoccupied with the implications of the event for themselves. Therefore, the first question to address is: How is the patient doing right now and are all the medical issues receiving the full attention they deserve?

- *Ensure that key individuals are notified and involved as soon as possible, including the attending physician and the hospital risk manager.*

  How far communication needs to go up the chain of command depends on the situation, the severity of the event, and the context. Since the cultural change we are trying to promote demands that transparency apply to all types of adverse events and medical error, disclosure should become standard practice for small as well as devastating errors. If a nurse's workload causes a short delay in getting a patient the next dose of a pain medication, a simple explanation and apology to the patient may be sufficient, without involving or notifying anyone else. However, clinicians need to be cognizant of which errors require prompt reporting (even on nights or weekends) as well as those that should be communicated at once to hospital leaders for their immediate attention.

- *Contact a designated "coach" and make arrangements for a meeting to plan disclosure.*

  Again, while some events can certainly be managed by a simple and straightforward explanation to the patient, events that will have a significant effect on a patient's care or outcome generally require thoughtful deliberation and planning with a knowledgeable and experienced consultant, or "coach."

  While some health care organizations may choose to give coaches decisional authority in these situations, most seem to prefer a model that sees the coach in much the same role as a medical consultant. In other words, the role of the coach is to provide support, practical advice, and the informed perspective of someone who is not directly involved in the event. Serious disagreements about whether disclosure should occur, or about the information that should be communicated, should be rare but may require further discussions up the institutional chain of command.

  Physicians often assume that since they are the ones with primary responsibility for the overall care of the patient, they are therefore the only ones that need to be involved in these conversations. Both the literature and our experience, however, support the view that since almost all medical errors involve more than just one clinician, coaches should represent a cross-section of professional disciplines. Likewise, all members of the team should be involved in planning and carrying out disclosure communication with the patient and family.

- *If the adverse event involved medical equipment or devices, ensure that these have been sequestered for later investigation.*

  Clinicians will likely want to contact their hospital risk manager for advice about how to properly sequester items for review and investigation.

- *Approach clinicians collaboratively and use the ask-tell-ask method.*

  Coaches can convey a collaborative approach by *asking* clinicians what they understand about the event that has occurred, *telling* them additional, targeted information in a way that incorporates the clinicians' current understanding and is comprehensible to them, and then *asking* how they understand and feel about the information that has been given.

  For example, the coach, after hearing the details of an event, might *ask*: "Do we have a consensus that this was clearly an error on the part of the team?" If the response is affirmative, the coach might then *tell*: "Based on what I am hearing, it seems clear we made an error for which we are responsible. In addition to giving a clear explanation to the patient and family about what happened, I think we need to apologize." Depending on the response of the clinicians, the coach might then *ask*, "How do all of you feel about making an apology? Who should apologize? At what point in the conversation do you think the apology should be made?"

  Coaches can also help clinicians by reminding them to see the disclosure conversation with the patient and family as a collaborative, back-and-forth process. Coaches can suggest that clinicians themselves use the ask-tell-ask method as a way of keeping the conversation interactive. When appropriate, coaches can provide a concrete example and invite clinicians to role-play the use of the approach as a means of preparing.

- *Gather information about the event from all the clinicians involved.*

  A good first step is to obtain as much information as possible from everyone who was involved. For more complex or serious events, this is usually best accomplished through a small team meeting or "huddle." In less complicated situations, of course, more informal ways of information gathering may be appropriate.

- *Determine whether the adverse event meets the threshold requiring disclosure to the patient or family.*

  Two useful rules of thumb are that an event should be disclosed if, first, it may result in a change in medical treatment for the patient, now or in the future or, second, you would want to know about the event if it happened to you or a member of your family. At a more practical level, it is also prudent to disclose any adverse events that are documented in the chart, since patients and families have full legal access to the medical record and failure to discuss events described in the chart could be seen as an attempt to minimize or even conceal them.

  While this approach makes sense, it does have some pitfalls. For example, the clinicians may feel that the error was trivial because it did not have a significant impact on the patient's course or outcome and may reason that, since it would not be important to them as clinicians, they have no obligation to disclose it to the patient. In these situations it is especially important to try to understand the situation from the perspective of the patient and to appreciate that patients may see some types of events as more significant than they are viewed by the clinicians.

  Events that are "near misses" are frequently a source of debate. On the one hand, disclosure of some near misses may provide no benefit and only serve to increase the patient's fears and anxieties. On the other hand, particularly when a patient may have been aware that something happened that was not routine or was out of the ordinary, disclosure may be imperative in order to maintain trust and avoid creating the impression that a secret is being kept from the patient.

- *Remind the team that this conversation is for the benefit of the patient and family and that the needs of clinicians will be addressed separately.*

  Adverse events and medical errors prompt a long list of important considerations ranging from the immediate care of the patient to performing a root cause analysis and developing a strategy for improvement. Clinicians need to remember, however, that the agenda for the initial meeting with the patient and family is solely to provide them with the information and support they need. Clinicians should be careful not to use this meeting as an opportunity to assign blame, vent frustrations, or promote their own interests.

Coaches or clinical leaders can play a critical role here by helping the team to prepare a unified message for the family and by soliciting agreement that the clinicians will not use this conversation as an opportunity for debating the facts or for parsing responsibility. It may be helpful to be explicit on this point—"I know how difficult this is for everyone and that there are lots of strong feelings, but the purpose of this meeting is to support the patient and family, not to iron out the disagreements or assign blame."

- *Determine which clinicians should be present for the initial conversation.*

  As a rule of thumb, all the key clinicians who were involved in the event should be invited to participate in the meeting with the patient and family. Exceptions to this rule of thumb should be considered when there is reason to believe that the family would find a meeting with several clinicians intimidating or threatening, when members of the clinical team are too angry or self-absorbed to be able to participate in the meeting as team players, or when a clinician is too emotionally distraught to make a productive contribution. When it fits the situation, consider involving clinical leaders, like division chiefs or nurse managers, to serve as support for more junior clinicians. The hospital risk manager or others who are not clinically involved should usually *not* participate in this initial meeting, as this can send a misleading message to the patient and family.

- *Assess who should be present for support of the patient and family.*

  At times of stress, patients and family members can be strengthened by having a network of support around themselves. Clinicians can support this process by prompting the family to identify individuals who might be helpful, such as friends, family members, primary care providers, or clergy. Hospital social workers can be very helpful in contacting these individuals and facilitating their involvement in these meetings. If English is not the patient's primary language, an interpreter may be needed. Even families who may speak English well enough to communicate in routine health care situations may benefit from an interpreter, given the inherent level of stress in this kind of conversation.

- *Decide who should lead the conversation.*

  In most situations, patients and families will prefer to hear bad news from a clinician with whom they have an established relationship. Most often this will be the attending physician, but in certain cases it might be a nurse or a community physician who has a good perspective on the overall care of the patient. While in some situations there may be an important role for members of the hospital leadership to take in these conversations, families in the immediate aftermath of a serious event are reassured when they experience continuity in their clinical care and a sense of commitment and accountability on the part of their primary caregivers.
- *Agree on the core information that will be communicated.*

  A critical element of the planning process is for the clinical team to come to clear agreement about the core content of the information they are going to share with the patient and family, even if they are not directly asked. As noted below, this should include all the facts that are known at that time and should not include speculation. Second, the team should anticipate questions the patient or family may ask and formulate answers that will be responsive to the expressed concerns without going beyond the facts as they are known at that moment.

  Finally, coaches should consider encouraging the clinical team to practice some of this communication ahead of time, such as by role-playing different scenarios with the coach in the role of the patient. This can be very helpful in giving those involved a chance to put their thoughts and feelings into words and minimize the chance that they will stumble or stray into unhelpful territory during the conversation itself.

- *Determine an optimal time and setting for the conversation.*

  A common dilemma for clinicians is whether to have a conversation with the family promptly, when little is known about the details of the event, or to wait, even a matter of hours, until more information can be obtained. In general, an initial conversation should occur very early, within the first few hours if possible and nearly always within the first 24 hours. Responding in a timely manner conveys seriousness and a relational commitment to the patient and family and avoids giving the impression that the team is "buying time" to cover up the event. One implication of having a conversation early, however, is that there are likely to be fewer facts available. In this context, clinicians should communicate what is known so far and offer reassurance that more information will be shared as it becomes known.

  As with any difficult conversation in health care, location is important. Sometimes a conversation at the bedside will be necessary in order to accommodate the patient's participation in the conversation. Otherwise, a quiet location away from the bedside, where everyone can be comfortably seated, is ideal. Clinicians should remember to turn off their pagers and arrange for clinical coverage for the duration of the meeting.

- *Decide who will take primary responsibility for following up, so that this can be communicated unambiguously to the family.*

  In these early conversations, clinicians are in the position of responding to a rupture in their relationship with the patient and family and of attempting to rebuild trust at a time when it is likely to be fragile and threatened. It is therefore imperative for the clinicians to convey their accountability and promote as much continuity and appropriate follow-through as possible. This can include such actions as ensuring that pertinent information is located and shared, that follow-up meetings are kept on time, and that those who say they will attend actually do so.

- *Discuss with the team how the patient's culture, health literacy, disabilities, and level of sedation may impact the conversation.*

  Explicit discussion of the communication needs and preferences of the patient and family prior to the meeting can be helpful. Understanding the cognitive capacities of the patient and family, as well as choosing the right emotional tone for the conversation, are essential. Families can feel disrespected by clinicians who assume too much medical knowledge or who use medical jargon, but they can also be offended by clinicians who overly simplify the clinical reality or talk down to them.

Patients and family members who are angry may not respond well to clinicians who are emotionally solicitous and may benefit from a more reserved demeanor, at least until some trust has been restored. Clinicians should be prepared for responses from the patient and family that may at other times be out of character, such as overt sadness, sarcastic anger, or impassivity. When there is reason to be concerned about the potential for violence, clinicians should take appropriate precautions, such as choosing an appropriate location for the meeting and involving security personnel as indicated.

The Conversation with the Patient and Family

- *Bring your own caring and humanness to the conversation.*

  Communicating with patients and families in the aftermath of adverse events and error does not require clinicians to master a completely new set of communication skills. Clinicians are well served by recognizing that these conversations will be most successful when they are understood as one version of the kinds of honest, caring, and compassionate conversations physicians have daily with patients and family members.

  In this context, each person has different styles, strengths, and weaknesses in the ways they interact with patients and families. Coaches and clinical leaders can help clinicians by encouraging them to be themselves, helping them to build on the strengths that they bring to interpersonal relationships. At the same time, clinicians must recognize that in these situations patients and families need clinicians to be authentic and genuine in their efforts to connect.

- *Remember the core relational values that can help to rebuild relationships when trust has been ruptured.*

  Clinicians should remember that trust is the sine qua non of their relationships with patients and families and that a serious adverse event or medical error is likely to rupture that trust. By striving to live up to core relational values—transparency, respect, accountability, continuity, and kindness—as they engage with the patient and family, they can take a concrete step towards rebuilding that trust.

- *Apply the "Golden Rule": What would you want to be told if you were the patient?*

  As noted above, one of the most difficult issues in preparing for these conversations is deciding how much to tell patients and families about what happened. Multiple and competing considerations are at play in this decision, but again it is often helpful to refer to a very simple but compelling principle—the "Golden Rule" of treating others as you would like to be treated. The pitfall of this approach is, of course, that sometimes the preferences and desires of the patient and family members are not necessarily the same as those of the clinicians. Nonetheless, this is generally a good place to start and can serve as a reminder that these conversations are, first and foremost, opportunities to treat patients and families with respect.

- *Convey compassion and empathy for the patient's and family's suffering.*

  Surveys of family members show that one of their most important—and frequently unmet—needs is to have their pain and suffering acknowledged by clinicians. In addition to putting kindness into action by conveying compassion and empathy, it can be helpful to use words to express one's effort to acknowledge and validate the suffering of the patient and family. Words like "We are so sorry that this has happened," "This must be a nightmare for you," or "I can't imagine how hard this must be for you" can help to begin the process of re-building trust.

- *Set the agenda for the meeting.*

  The initial conversation after an adverse event or error can be very intimidating for patients and family members. After what has probably involved routine clinical care and many informal conversations with various caregivers, suddenly an event has occurred that has led to a much more formal conversation with their attending and numerous other clinicians, some of whom they may barely know. Clinicians may incorrectly assume that the patient and family are aware of the purpose of the meeting, leading to confusion and perhaps unmet expectations. The person leading the conversation should therefore remember to begin by setting out why this meeting is taking place, the agenda for the meeting, and the goals that the team hopes to achieve. This person should then be sure to check in with the family and confirm that this agenda is acceptable to them and meets their needs, or solicit and include other issues that the family would like to have addressed.

- *Communicate collaboratively by using the ask-tell-ask method.*

  Clinicians may be tempted to respond to emotion or awkward silences by providing a lengthy monologue to the patient and family about the clinical facts of what happened and what will be done to prevent problems from recurring in the future. While there is certainly essential information that should be communicated following an error, a key challenge is to ensure that the disclosure is customized to the needs and preferences of the particular patient and family. In order to customize the conversation, there needs to be ample back-and-forth communication. The ask-tell-ask method can help to facilitate this interactivity.

  For example the clinician might *ask*, "It would be helpful for me to hear your understanding of what happened today—can you tell me?" After hearing the response, the clinician might then *tell*, "Yes, you're right, there was an overdose of medication, but there's some additional information I want to share with you." Then, based on the response, the clinician might *ask* questions such as, "Can you help me determine whether I communicated clearly by telling me what you heard me say?"; "Do you have any questions for me about what happened today?"; and "How are you feeling about what's happened—what can we do to make you feel more comfortable?"

- *Clearly state the facts as they are known at the present.*

  A guiding principle behind all discussions with patients and families is that there is never any legal risk to disclosing all facts as they are known at the present. Indeed, in legal proceedings facts inevitably become known, and it is almost always to the advantage of clinicians if they are known sooner rather than later. This being said, the problem and the peril is in knowing what counts as a "fact."

  Good clinicians have been trained in how to take a relatively small number of facts—from the history, physical, and laboratory data—and make a complete story about why a patient is ill. In many ways, this is the essence of being a good diagnostician. In the context of an adverse event, however, this strength has the potential to become a liability. Whereas patients are generally quite tolerant of clinical plans that change in response to new information, they can become fixed on the first explanation that is offered following an adverse event or error. Then, when the story changes in light of new information, they can interpret the change as an attempt to cover up the truth or to avoid responsibility. This is why clinicians do need to modify their communication style in this context, being more perspicacious and cautious in the way that they connect the dots and extrapolate from limited information to the big picture. Risk managers warn that the first explanations of adverse events are frequently incomplete and sometimes completely wrong. One of the most important tasks before meeting with the patient and family is therefore to come to agreement on what are the known "facts" of the case and what observations are better defined as speculation and conjecture and in need of further clarification.

  One insight that some clinicians find helpful is to remember that patients want to hear an explanation that enables them to make sense of what has happened and of their current situation. For example, while patients and families can generally understand that all the facts may not be immediately available at the first conversation, they will likely be much less tolerant and understanding if it appears that facts that *are* known are being withheld from them or if basic data like lab values and x-ray results are still "missing" or "unknown" several days after the event.

- *Consider whether this is one of the rare circumstances in which disclosure of the facts may not be of immediate benefit to the patient/family.*

  A long-recognized exception to the principle of truth telling in medicine is the "therapeutic exception," which states that clinicians may withhold information from patients when disclosure would be harmful to them. As understood in ethics and law, this principle should be interpreted very narrowly and cautiously, particularly in the context of adverse events and error. The picture is further complicated by the fact that in these situations clinicians are often motivated to find ways to avoid having these very difficult conversations with patients and families, and the "therapeutic exception" can become a convenient and welcome excuse for not doing so. As a rule of thumb, therefore, clinicians should be committed to disclosure as soon as the patient and family are capable of having the conversation. Decisions to the contrary must meet a very high threshold of justification; indeed, one hospital's disclosure policy explicitly requires consultation from an ethics committee before clinicians can choose not to disclose.

- *Convey caring always, and apologize when appropriate.*

  Human societies have developed exceptionally complex systems for expressions of apology and regret, with their attendant expectations of compensation and forgiveness. Unfortunately, much of the rhetoric surrounding medical error has focused on the simple phrase "I'm sorry." While everyone has learned at a young age from parents and teachers the power of this phrase in resolving disputes following accidents on the playground, it does not fully capture the complexities that often exist in the clinical world.

  The subtleties of this issue were discussed above in more detail, but some commonsense distinctions may be helpful here.

Expressions of empathy and compassion for what the patient is experiencing are always appropriate ("I am so sorry this happened to you"). However, expressions of personal or institutional responsibility for an adverse event should also be made when the facts indicate that the event was an avoidable consequence of a medical error. While clinicians may feel somewhat psychologically cleansed by telling a patient that "this was our fault and we are so sorry," it is in fact unwarranted—and unethical—to accept such responsibility on behalf of oneself and others when the facts have not yet shown it to be true.

- *Explain what is being done to care for the patient and the plan for care going forward.*

  In keeping with the principle that the first and most important consideration following an adverse event is the care of the patient, clinicians should be reminded to review the current situation with the patient and family and to assure them that care will go forward as seamlessly as possible.

- *Assess whether the existing clinical relationships can be maintained or whether care needs to be transitioned to alternative providers.*

  While patients always have the right to request transfer to alternative care providers or institutions, in the immediate aftermath of an adverse event this may not be in the patient's best interest. Therefore clinicians should generally seek ways to work with patients and families to restore and maintain trust and to sustain clinical continuity. Sometimes it may be helpful and sufficient to offer the family a second opinion or the involvement of additional subspecialists to obtain other clinical insights or to reassure the patient and family that the care is on track.

- *Assure the patient/family that the event will be thoroughly investigated and that all facts will be communicated as they become known.*

  One of the challenges of an institutional commitment to early disclosure of adverse events and errors is that clinicians will often have to tell patients and families that little is known at the time of the initial conversation and that most of the information and explanation will have to await the collection of further data. This may be difficult for the family to accept, but clinicians need to be prepared to resist the pressure to come up with premature explanations that "put it all together." Instead, they should focus on reassuring the family that the investigation will be prompt and thorough and that if it reveals that mistakes were made, these will be fully disclosed. In addition, clinicians can assure patients and families that the institution will respond to any errors that are identified with steps to minimize the risk of such events in the future and that the hospital will follow up with families to inform them of the details of these safety improvements if desired. Some organizations are making explicit commitments to conducting accelerated root cause analyses, decreasing the length of time families would need to wait for information about what caused the event in question.[139]

- *Acknowledge that questions about financial compensation are appropriate and legitimate and that they will be addressed by others with the qualifications and authority to do so.*

  Clinicians are often concerned that the family will ask about financial issues, such as whether the hospital will cover the additional expenses associated with an adverse event or error, whether they can have vouchers for travel, food, or lodging, or whether the hospital is going to compensate them directly for the injury. Clinicians may feel compelled to accede to these requests as an expression of goodwill or compassion. Clinicians need to anticipate these questions and be prepared to resist responding directly to these requests, unless they have the authority to do so, since some may have consequences for the clinicians involved and for the institution that cannot be immediately foreseen or honored.

  Clinicians should respond to these requests by acknowledging to the patient and family that they are appropriate and legitimate questions and that they will be addressed by someone from the hospital with the proper qualifications and authority. These questions should be promptly communicated to those in the risk management department so that they can respond directly to the family in a timely fashion. In particular, since hospitals now often have mechanisms for generating bills to patients and third-party payers almost immediately after services are provided, the hospital may want to develop a strategy for delaying the generation of those bills until additional information can be gathered and obtained.

- *Offer support services—chaplains, social workers, patient advocates.*

  While the initial conversation generally includes those who have an existing clinical relationship with the patient, clinicians should emphasize that the hospital has many other resources available for those who have experienced an adverse event or error, including chaplains, social workers, and patient advocates. The clinicians should offer to contact these individuals and enlist their help if desired. An important additional resource is the organization Medically Induced Trauma Support Services (MITSS), available through its Web site, www.mitss.org/.

  As noted above, an important element of rebuilding and maintaining trust is making plans for follow-up and then being sure that this follow-up occurs. At the end of the conversation, therefore, a plan for future meetings should be explicitly discussed. Finally, in keeping with the needs of families for recognition of what they are going through, the clinicians should close the meeting with a compassionate expression of concern for the pain and suffering of the patient and family, regardless of whether these are the result of an error.

- *Remember that disclosure may not be greeted with thanks or forgiveness.*

  When the situation calls for an apology, clinicians may experience tremendous relief and healing from an opportunity to express their regret and remorse to the patient directly. Clinicians, however, may be hoping for an expression of forgiveness from the patient or family, feeling that resolution will not be complete unless this happens.

  Often, however, patients and their families will not be prepared to forgive at the time of the initial conversation, and sometimes they will not be inclined to forgive at any point in time. This can create the potential for the clinician to feel even worse, having shown vulnerability through the act of apologizing without receiving the reassurance that comes from the reciprocal act of forgiveness. This psychological dynamic will be unavoidable in many of these difficult conversations; therefore, clinicians may benefit from being prepared for how unmet expectations for forgiveness may affect them emotionally.

Documentation and Follow-up

- *Debrief the event, whenever possible, with a postconversation huddle.*

  While the purpose of the conversation with the patient and family is solely to provide them with support, these conversations often generate new concerns and tensions within the clinical team, including uncertainty about responsibilities going forward, questions about the nature of the investigation into the event, and interpersonal tensions that inevitably arise over issues of causation and blame. Whenever possible, the clinicians should attempt to meet together after the conversation, ideally with a coach or clinical leader, to debrief the event.

- *Assess the emotional and psychological needs of the clinicians involved and ensure follow-up for clinicians impacted by the event.*

  The coach or a person in a position of clinical leadership should emphasize to the clinicians that feelings of anxiety, anger, and shame are normal and to be expected. Reassure those involved that clinicians in this situation are routinely provided resources for support and that support does not in any way imply poor coping or an inability to handle the situation. Again, the organization MITSS may be a helpful resource and can be contacted at www.mitss.org/.

- *Document the conversation in the medical record.*

  The medical record should include a summary of the initial meeting with the patient and family, including a summary of the facts surrounding the adverse event, a synopsis of the initial conversation (including a list of those present), and a description of the care provided and current plans for care going forward.

- *Do not document the coaching intervention in the medical record.*

  For institutions that have adopted a formal coaching model, such as that recommended by the NQF, there may be a question as to whether advice from the coach should be documented in the medical record. Our recommendation is that this advice should not appear in the record. The rationale for this is grounded in the fact that the patient's chart is a record of the patient's treatment and the interactions between the clinicians and the patient. Since the purpose of the coach is to provide support, information, and counseling for the staff, the subject and content of those conversations do not belong in the patient's medical record.

EIGHT

Learning through Enacting

After coaches and clinicians have been exposed to the core relational values, knowledge base, and just-in-time guidelines for the practice of disclosure, it is important to have an opportunity to see practice in action and then to reflect on that practice. In our workshops, we aim to achieve depth by enacting one paradigmatic case in detail and breadth by discussing a wide range of cases in a briefer format. The paradigmatic case is not based on an actual event, but rather was developed to constitute a realistic scenario—a medication error leading to a respiratory arrest—that would be familiar and accessible to practitioners from a variety of backgrounds, specialties, and professional disciplines. Below, we present a narrative description of the case scenario and summarize several representative ways that the case has been approached by different participants.

We emphasize at the outset that the purpose of the enactment is not to label certain approaches as good and others as bad. Rather, we think of the scenario, the actors, and the volunteer participants as coming together at each workshop to produce a unique "moment" of clinical practice, which participants can reflect on, individually and collectively, to deepen their knowledge and skill base for addressing the issues that emerge.

Professional actors are in the roles of the patient and her husband. Before each workshop, we select a participant to play the role of coach, based on who will be attending the workshop. Normally, we choose a clinician who has been playing this role informally in the organization already and is therefore likely to have credibility with the group and to be sufficiently comfortable taking on the coaching role.

In these situations, an important early step is for the coach to organize a "huddle" of the key clinical participants to review what has happened and prepare for the first conversation with the patient and family. Therefore, we ask the coach whom he or she would like to include in the huddle. Invariably, the coach requests the involvement of the patient's attending, the surgical intern, and the bedside nurse. In addition, some coaches have requested inclusion of the nurse manager of the unit, a social worker, or a chaplain. Participants are then asked to volunteer for each of these roles. We generally ask that each role be filled by a person from the corresponding professional background (e.g., nurses in the role of nurses), as this helps to ensure that the enactment will be experienced as realistic. In addition, we ask volunteers in the coaching and disclosure enactments to respond as they would in real life.

The enactment is then carried out at the front of the room, in two parts. For the first 10 to 15 minutes, the coach meets with the clinicians who have been identified to be part of the huddle. In this conversation, the coach faces a complex set of tasks. In a short period of time, the coach needs to assess the emotional state of those who were involved in the event (Are any of the clinicians too angry or upset to participate? Are they capable of being team players in the meeting with the patient and family?). In addition to determining which of the clinicians will meet and speak with the patient and family, the coach must help the team develop an agenda for the conversation and formulate a plan for what they will be told (What are the facts that we can and should share at this time? Are there areas of uncertainty where we should avoid conjecture and speculation? Is it fitting in this situation to apologize?). The coach needs to help the team anticipate difficult questions that might be raised by the patient or family member ("Who will pay for the extra costs associated with this event?" "What if I don't want that nurse taking care of me anymore?")

Once the coach feels the team has been adequately prepared for the conversation, we take a short break in the workshop while the scene is set for the second conversation, which takes place at the patient's bedside. The patient is in a hospital gown, attached to an IV, with her husband seated beside her. The clinicians are given the cue to join them, and the initial disclosure conversation takes place. Our approach is improvisational—the flow and content of the conversation emerges naturally from the nature of the unique interactions in each enactment. In this way, our approach to learning differs markedly from the method employed with "standardized patients," in which actors typically operate within defined scripts. In our enactments, when the actors experience the clinicians as honest and caring, they tend to feel reassured and open to a process in which the relationships that have been ruptured can begin to be repaired. When they feel the clinicians are concealing information or less than authentic, they are likely to become more anxious, irritable, and demanding.

The Case of Brigid O'Malley

The hypothetical case we use is that of Mrs. Brigid O'Malley, an otherwise healthy 45-year-old woman who is admitted to the hospital's oncology ward following an exploratory laparotomy and lysis of adhesions for a small bowel obstruction. She has a history of colon cancer, which was successfully treated with surgical resection and chemotherapy two years ago, and she is now thought to be in remission.

Dr. Alan Jones, the surgical intern, has written postoperative orders, a portion of which are shown in figure 5. Of note, he has written an order for the patient to be started on PCA (patient-controlled analgesia, a technique that allows patients to control their pain by self-administering morphine or other analgesics by pushing a button connected to an infusion pump). Since these devices must be prepared by the pharmacy, the intern orders a continuous infusion of morphine for the patient, at a dose of 5.0 mg/hr, to be administered in the interim.

When the nurse reads the morphine order, she does not notice the decimal point. She asks Dr. Jones why he wrote for so much morphine; he replies that the patient seems to have a high tolerance for opioids and that she required multiple boluses in the PACU (i.e., recovery room) before coming back to the ward. The nurse, Ms. Diane Sutton, begins the infusion at 50 mg/hr at about noon. Three hours later, she responds to an alarm from the room and finds the patient apneic, bradycardic, and with a low oxygen saturation. She calls a code and initiates mask ventilation. The code team responds; they find the patient apneic but not pulseless. When it becomes evident that the patient is on a morphine infusion, the team leader stops the infusion and orders naloxone, 400 mcg IV. The

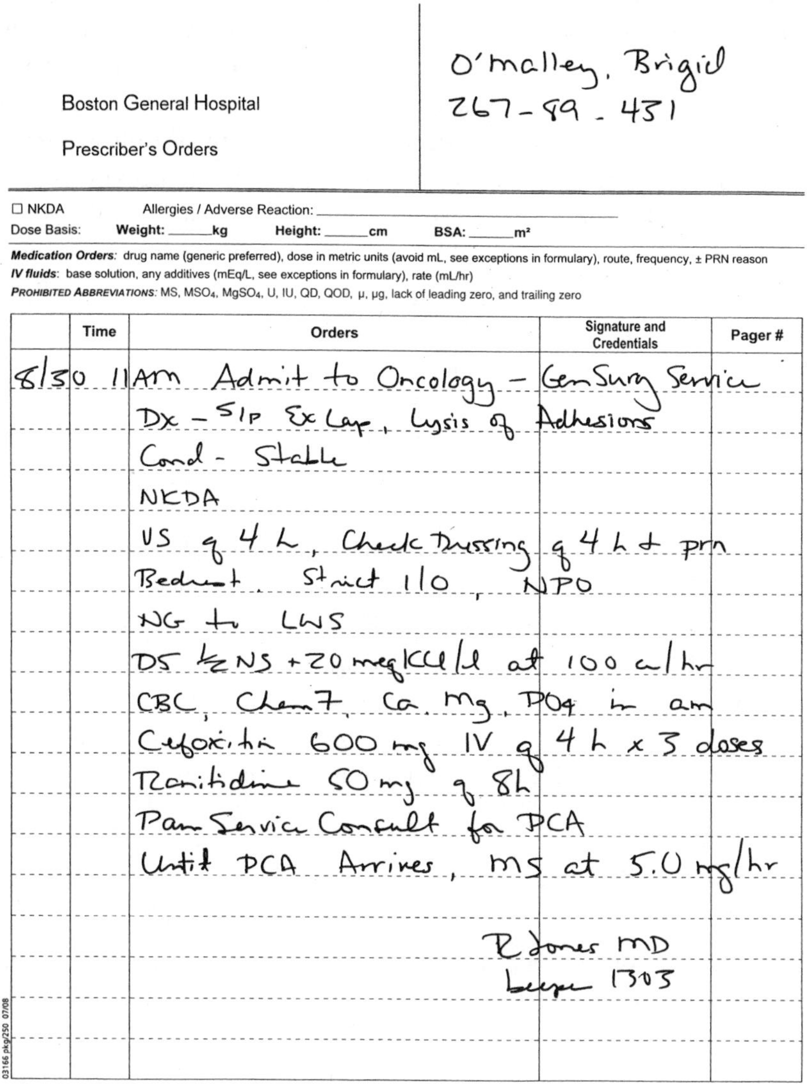

Boston General Hospital

Prescriber's Orders

O'Malley, Brigid
267-99-431

☐ NKDA Allergies / Adverse Reaction: ______

Dose Basis: **Weight:** ______kg **Height:** ______cm **BSA:** ______m²

***Medication Orders**:* drug name (generic preferred), dose in metric units (avoid mL, see exceptions in formulary), route, frequency, ± PRN reason
***IV fluids**:* base solution, any additives (mEq/L, see exceptions in formulary), rate (mL/hr)
***PROHIBITED ABBREVIATIONS**:* MS, MSO4, MgSO4, U, IU, QD, QOD, μ, μg, lack of leading zero, and trailing zero

	Time	Orders	Signature and Credentials	Pager #
8/30	11AM	Admit to Oncology – Gen Surg Service		
		Dx – S/P Ex Lap, Lysis of Adhesions		
		Cond – Stable		
		NKDA		
		VS q 4 h, Check Dressing q 4 h + prn		
		Bedrest, Strict I/O, NPO		
		NG to LWS		
		D5 ½NS + 20 meq KCl/l at 100 cc/hr		
		CBC, Chem 7, Ca, Mg, PO4 in am		
		Cefoxitin 600 mg IV q 4 h x 3 doses		
		Ranitidine 50 mg q 8h		
		Pain Service Consult for PCA		
		Until PCA Arrives, MS at 5.0 mg/hr		
		R Jones MD		
		Beeper 1303		

03166 pkg/250 07/08

FIGURE 5. The case of Brigid O'Malley

patient responds, begins to breathe on her own, and is transferred to the ICU for monitoring and observation.

While the surgical house officer believes he wrote the order correctly, the nurse does not feel that she is entirely to blame. As shown in figure 5, Dr. Jones wrote the order with a "trailing zero" (i.e., as 5.0 mg/hr instead of as 5 mg/hr), which is prohibited by hospital policy precisely to prevent this type of error. Given the incorrect format of the order, the nurse was not primed to "see" the decimal point. Furthermore, the nurse had been appropriately assertive by questioning the order and was given reassurance that the patient needed a larger dose than normal. Unfortunately, while the nurse thought she was questioning why Dr. Jones had written for 50 mg/hr, Dr. Jones thought she was questioning why he had written an order for 5 mg/hr—a critical breakdown in communication. Furthermore, although an order for a morphine infusion at 50 mg/hr would automatically trigger review in many clinical settings, doses this high are occasionally necessary for oncology patients, reducing the nurse's level of concern about implementing the order. Finally, the pharmacy may have contributed to the communication breakdown, since doses of this magnitude are often challenged and investigated by the pharmacist before being dispensed.

By early that evening, Mrs. O'Malley is doing well, sitting up in a chair. She is expected to make a full recovery. Bill O'Malley, her husband, is with her at the bedside. The couple has been told that the patient's attending physician will stop by soon to discuss the events of the afternoon and to answer their questions. The attending and the hospital coach have both been notified of the event, and the coach has requested a brief meeting with those who were involved to discuss the incident.

Paths and Pitfalls

Below we discuss five representative ways in which the clinical teams in our workshops have approached the challenge of communicating this event to Brigid O'Malley and her husband. Each approach provides a realistic example on which the participants in the workshop can reflect and from which everyone can learn.

"Just the facts, ma'am"

A central guideline that we emphasize to workshop participants is that they should always be willing to share known facts with the patient and family. Stated more strongly, there is rarely a good reason not to share whatever facts are known, as soon as they are known. That said, it can be quite challenging to identify what counts as a fact (which can and should be shared) and what counts as speculation (which should generally not be immediately discussed). In the many workshops we have conducted, coaches and clinical teams have arrived at radically different conclusions about what counts as a "fact" in this case. At one end of the spectrum, clinicians have shared a great deal of information, explaining meticulously how the event was the result of a "perfect storm" of errors, including the use of the "trailing zero," the failure of the nurse to read the order correctly, the failure of the nurse and intern to communicate clearly about whether the dose was appropriate, and the failure of the pharmacy to double-check the order before filling it. Other teams have shared some information, but with fewer details, such as revealing only that there was a "miscommunication" between the intern and the nurse. Still others have taken an even more cautious approach, insisting that virtually nothing could be known for sure so soon after the event. For example, one team told the family that an investigation would be performed and the team would report back after the investigation was complete but that until the infusion pump was dismantled and the gears examined for possible malfunction, nothing could be said with any certainty about why the error had happened.

"It was all his/her/their fault"

One of the deepest traits in human nature is the impulse to find someone to blame when something goes wrong. The act of blaming allows those involved to have a sense that they understand how and why the error occurred, and it provides a rationale for punishment and a claim for recompense. As discussed above, however, medical errors are rarely the result of the isolated failure of an individual. Most often they occur when a series of small and latent errors or conditions come into alignment. In these situations, individuals who appear to be responsible are very often as much "victims" of the error as they are the "villains" who made it happen. In this sense, the act of blaming leads to a mistaken understanding of the event, resulting in the false assumption that assigning blame and punishing or eliminating the person who is seen as responsible will prevent the error from occurring in the future.

Despite a more nuanced understanding of the ecology of mistakes in medical settings, the tendency to blame remains strong. In one workshop, the attending physician stated that he wanted to meet with the patient and her husband alone. The coach for the session tried to dissuade him from doing so, pointing out that the intern and the nurse involved were both willing and even motivated to attend the meeting. The attending persisted, however, and ultimately the coach and the other participants gave in to his wishes.

When he met with the patient and her husband, the attending's strategy became more clear. Although he began the conversation by stating that he was totally responsible for everything that happened during the patient's stay in the hospital, he quickly added that the hospital is designed to run on a system of trainees and that the shortage of nurses had forced the hospital to hire young and inexperienced nurses. Unfortunately, he went on to explain, this trainee physician and inexperienced nurse were responsible for the serious error that occurred. He promised the patient and her husband that these young clinicians would be held responsible for the event and that he would do whatever he could to see that nothing like this happened again.

In other workshops, the decision is made in the huddle that either the intern or the nurse should not be present for the conversation. The intern may come across as too defensive or accusatory, or the nurse may appear too vulnerable or intimidated, to be seen as productive participants in the imminent conversation. Although it never seems to be the intention of clinicians when they talk with the patient and her husband, we have observed that the one who is not present tends to emerge in the conversation as most culpable, regardless of the actual circumstances surrounding the error.

Despite continuous efforts to encourage clinicians to see that most medical errors are the result of flawed systems of care, the culture of blame persists as a powerful force, especially when one or more of the parties involved is not included in the initial discussion of the event, the conversations that follow with the patient and family, or any debriefing among clinicians afterward. A commitment to include all of the involved parties in the disclosure process can serve as a strong countervailing force to the powerful tendency to blame.

"It was all my fault"

Just as the culture of medicine has been slow to relinquish a tendency to blame, so have individual clinicians continued to view the acceptance of blame as a virtue. It is not uncommon to hear examples of the senior and experienced attending surgeon who stands up at a Morbidity and Mortality (M&M) conference and announces in front of all of her peers that the error under discussion is entirely of her doing and that she takes full and unmitigated responsibility. Confessions like this appear heroic, and younger clinicians tend to see these clinicians as role models. At the same time, clinicians with less power may accept blame as an expression of their perceived or actual lack of status in the hierarchy.

We have seen this latter example play out in several of our workshops, when the bedside nurse involved in the medication error verbalizes during the coaching session: "It was all my fault . . . I should have seen the decimal point . . . I could have questioned the intern more definitively . . . I should have realized this was an inappropriate dose." Despite the fact that the "truth" of the matter is far more complex, there can be a tendency within the clinician group to accept this confession and to consider the matter resolved. In addition to possibly exposing this individual inappropriately to professional censure or legal liability, the failure to appreciate the complexity of the error makes it unlikely that corrective action will be taken to prevent similar events in the future.

"All's well that ends well"

Everyone, of course, wants to hear good news, and clinicians and patients alike are generally relieved and gratified when a potentially serious incident turns out to have not caused serious medical harm. Thus some of the attendings who have participated in our workshops have focused on this aspect of the event in explaining what occurred to the patient and her husband. One physician noted: "Unfortunately, you received the wrong dose of a medication, but it was promptly recognized, you were treated appropriately, and you're going to be just fine." As the patient and her husband pressed him for more details, the attending persisted that, since everything turned out fine, there was little reason to be concerned about the details.

Although this can be a tempting strategy for clinicians, it fails to acknowledge the emotional trauma that is frequently inherent in this kind of event, even when the medical outcome is positive. In one workshop when this approach was used, the patient's husband refused to be placated and felt provoked to push back, insisting that the attending acknowledge the life-threatening nature of the event. Just because everything turned out "fine" this time, what assurance could they have that an event like this would not happen again, but with less favorable results? This scenario taught the group that while reassurance can be an important part of what is communicated to patients in the aftermath of a medical error, patients and families may be left with the impression that the event is being glossed over and that the magnitude and significance of the event—from the patient's perspective—is not being fully acknowledged and appreciated.

"Your loss is our learning experience"

Certainly a profound breakthrough of the patient safety movement has been the shift toward a more enlightened perspective about errors in complex health care organizations, as well as the critical necessity of learning from them. The literature indicates that this kind of organizational learning matters deeply to patients as well; when medical errors happen, patients and families are concerned not only about their own welfare but also the welfare of others to whom a similar event could occur. Accordingly, patients are invested, generally speaking, in knowing what steps are being taken to decrease the possibility or likelihood that what happened to them will happen to others.

We have observed clinicians, perhaps as an outgrowth of this orientation toward learning from errors, move the conversation with the patient and family rather hastily toward an emphasis on learning from the mistake and making the systems changes necessary to prevent it in the future: "We want you and your husband to know that our institution is deeply committed to continually improving the quality and safety of our care. We take this very seriously and will be investigating what happened carefully so we can prevent these mistakes in the future." One clinician even delved into an extended explanation about the hospital's plans to introduce CPOE—computer physician order entry—as a way to emphasize to the patient and her husband the priority that the hospital was giving to this issue.

As in the approach that exemplified "all's well that ends well," this message can be reassuring for patients and families to hear at the appropriate time. However, moving to this theme too quickly runs the risk of ignoring the threat to health and safety that has just occurred and conveying the impression that the clinicians do not appreciate the traumatic nature of the experience as lived by the patient and family.

Lessons Learned

The enactment and in-depth investigation of this single case scenario has been instructive in at least two ways. First, the case has provided rich material for discussion and reflection, giving participants the opportunity to thoughtfully examine many of the complex issues inherent in the coaching process. Second, it has enabled the workshop facilitators to observe the same case scenario being played out with a variety of clinicians pursuing a wide array of approaches. Indeed, having watched the same case scenario enacted with the same actors on multiple occasions, each time with a new set of clinicians, we have been struck by the context-driven uniqueness of how each enactment unfolds.

It has been a rich learning experience for us as educators, affording us a more textured and nuanced understanding of the relational complexities and challenges embedded in the disclosure process. Our expanded appreciation for the determining effects of context in these disclosure conversations argues for an understanding of competence as something that is never entirely achieved but rather discovered anew in each situation. As we entertain what a "best practice" of disclosure might look like for coaches and clinicians in the coming years, we do not envision any kind of scripted intervention that should be applied in all situations but rather a flexible response that will play out differently in every context, even when the facts of the case appear to be exactly the same.

Through enactment of the scenarios and the facilitated discussions that follow, our workshop participants have reported insight and growth at many levels. First, they typically report an awareness of self-efficacy, as they learn that they are actually quite capable of being effective in these conversations. This realization creates a confidence that feeds back on itself and makes them even more skilled in this role. Second, many hear feedback about particular aspects of their style and demeanor that they find especially helpful, from certain phrases they may use to particular aspects of their body language. Some of the best feedback in this regard typically comes from the actors, who experience the clinician in their roles of patient and family members but who have permission to provide the types of feedback that actual patients and family members do not have.

Third and perhaps most important, all of our scenarios raise profound ethical dilemmas for the participants. Unlike the abstract and theoretical ethical dilemmas that are usually discussed in bioethics classes, such as deciding which patient should get the last ventilator or whether euthanasia is morally permissible, these ethical dilemmas are intensely personal and arise within the relationships among clinicians and between clinicians and patient. They concern principles of justice, fairness, and how human beings should treat each other when bad things happen.

When a medical error occurs, the experience of trust that is the foundation of an optimal working relationship between clinician and the patient—or between the interdisciplinary team and the patient—is ruptured, and the clinician or team is in the position of either taking steps to address the breach in trust or behaving in ways that can deepen the rupture. In addition, clinicians involved in these events quite often suffer a diminution of trust in themselves, their capabilities, and their working relationships with each other. We have described the core relational values of transparency, respect, accountability, continuity, and kindness that are grounded in the working bonds that exist among clinicians, patients, and family members. These values can contribute to morally appropriate action on the part of clinicians in the aftermath of a medical error, action that has the potential to alleviate ruptured trust. We aim to distinguish this focus on ethics in everyday practice from more abstract approaches taught in bioethics classes. A distinguishing characteristic of this more grounded focus is that the "right" approach to communicating with patients and families in the aftermath of medical errors cannot be deduced through abstract reasoning but must be discerned, and indeed enacted, within the conversations themselves.

NINE

The Broad Spectrum of Adverse Events and Medical Error

Adverse events and medical error occur across a broad spectrum, from those that involve little or no harm to those that are catastrophic. In this chapter we explore how cases vary across a range of variables, such as differences between the inpatient and outpatient settings and between medical, surgical, and psychiatric patients. These cases raise questions such as when is it preferable for a nurse to have the disclosure conversation and when is it clinically justified to withhold information about an error from a patient or family member. The vignettes explore the distinctions between adverse events due to clearly preventable errors, those that are linked to unpreventable complications, and those that involve risks that were disclosed to the patient but that likely could have been avoided had there not been a lapse in concentration.

Our approach to exploring these vignettes is drawn from well-established methods developed in the field of bioethics. A central problem in moral philosophy is how to reason from abstract general principles to specific cases. A similar problem exists in questions about disclosure of adverse events and medical error in that the general principles that have been developed by organizations to date do not provide much useful guidance for the range of varied and complex situations faced by clinicians in everyday practice. In bioethics, using a methodological approach known as casuistry, we identify particular cases in which we have a high degree of confidence about the right course of action. These serve as "anchors," or paradigmatic cases. We then examine the more ambiguous cases and consider the ways in which they are similar to or different from these paradigmatic cases. By "triangulating" between the problematic case and these anchor points, we can arrive at a way of proceeding that is ethically sound.

In this section, we again emphasize the importance of a set of foundational values: transparency, respect, accountability, continuity and kindness—TRACK. In many examples of medical error, these central values are in synch, and the alignment of values suggests a clear and ethically uncomplicated approach. In some cases, however, these principles can be in conflict. Consider, for example, a situation in which a man with an anxiety disorder is admitted for minor surgery. He is written for three doses of cephazolin during the postoperative period. Because of a transcription error, each dose is one gram instead of the prescribed dose of 500 mg. Both of these doses are within in the acceptable prescription range for this purpose, and the patient suffers no identifiable harm. Should the error be disclosed?

The value of transparency might lead a clinician toward disclosing the error, but the value of kindness might argue against it, especially if the clinician was convinced that this communication would likely cause the patient needless anxiety at an already stressful time. According to the casuistic approach described above, one could consider comparable cases in which the correct course of action seems to be clear and then triangulate from these to examine more ambiguous cases. So, for example, if the dosing error had been much larger or associated with complications, the value of transparency would clearly prevail. In contrast, if the patient had a paranoid personality along with the anxiety disorder, there might be a clear argument in favor of nondisclosure. Since the example above is somewhere in between these two paradigmatic cases, one needs to reason about whether this situation is more like the case of the serious overdose (arguing for disclosure) or more like the case of the patient struggling with paranoia (which would weigh in favor of nondisclosure). While the process of collectively reasoning about these cases never attains scientific precision, it does provide a practical and systematic approach for finding an appropriate course of action.

Unlike the field of bioethics, the practice of communicating about adverse events and errors is still in its developmental infancy, and while consensus can be reached regarding some types of cases, many others reside firmly in the gray zone. As organizations create structures for thoughtfully approaching and learning from these cases over time, they will develop a portfolio of experience that will serve as a reference guide for managing subsequent cases. Eventually, organizations should develop a measure of collective confidence about the right course of action for cases that at present seem hopelessly controversial. In a way, our discussion of the cases presented here is a first step in seeking to develop this consensus.

For purposes of discussing these vignettes, we will assume the clinician involved is seeking assistance and advice about whether and/or how to disclose an event to a patient. For those institutions that have developed a coaching model, this consultant would be the person in the coaching role. For those that do not have a formal structure to provide coaching support, this individual would likely be a trusted and experienced colleague.

Our discussion of the cases is drawn from our use of these vignettes in the workshops that we have performed throughout the system of Harvard teaching hospitals, where we have asked for volunteer participants to imagine that they are the coach on call for their organization on a particular evening. Their beeper goes off, and when they answer the page, a clinician on the other end of the phone tells them about the particular clinical situation and asks for advice. The volunteer coach then provides the best guidance he or she can for two or three minutes, at which time the case is opened to general discussion. Below we have summarized many of the thoughts, suggestions, and questions that have emerged from these discussions, including points where agreement was reached as well as others where consensus has not been possible.

CALL FROM AN INTERNIST

I'm in clinic today, and I am about to see a 48-year-old man in follow-up for an elevated PSA level. Two weeks ago at his annual visit I ordered it as part of his screening labs, and it came back at 25 ng/ml (normal < 4 ng/ml).

Before entering the examination room, I was flipping through his chart and saw in the lab printouts the result from the PSA I ordered at his routine visit last year, which was 20 ng/ml. I don't know how this happened, but I am sure I never saw this result. Should I mention this result from last year when I see him now? If so, what should I say about it?

DISCUSSION. This case generally strikes a chord with many of our physician participants, as delays in diagnosis are one of the more common grounds for malpractice suits. PSA results are notoriously unreliable, with studies showing false positive rates of about 75 percent. Moreover, a "negative" reading has about a 20 percent chance of being inaccurate. Although some participants have therefore suggested deferring the decision of whether to disclose until after it is clear whether or not the patient has cancer, there has generally been wide consensus that disclosure is the proper course of action. The debate has therefore centered around the best timing for disclosure.

Since the physician is literally moments from entering the room to see the patient, some have suggested deferring the disclosure conversation until the next visit. Factors supporting this approach are that very little information is known at this point; indeed, it is possible that the lab slip is mislabeled and does not belong to this patient at all. Moreover, the goal of this visit is to make important decisions about how to proceed with the work-up for the elevated PSA level. Discussion of a possible medical error could be very distracting and could prevent the patient from being able to fully engage in decision making, a process that is necessary regardless of what the PSA level was one year ago. Once more information is gained and once a plan has been set, at a future visit the issue of the delayed lab result could be discussed with the patient.

A different approach would be to disclose the lab result at this visit, perhaps after a plan for the work-up has been developed and agreed on. The physician could say something like, "There is something else I need to tell you. Before I came in the room today I noticed that the screening PSA level we performed last year was also elevated. I'm really sorry about this, I don't know why I didn't see it, and indeed at this time I can't even be sure that there wasn't an error in labeling the result such that it is not even yours. But in any case I wanted you to know this as soon as possible, and I will follow up and have more information for you the next time I see you." This approach has an important advantage. When the patient sees a urologist or other specialist, one of the first questions asked will be what the PSA levels have been in the past. If this physician looks them up in the medical record, the previously elevated level would likely be disclosed to the patient, without the internist having had a chance to explain the circumstances surrounding the event.

Finally, one practical suggestion came from a participant who suggested this might be a good time to request a favor from a urologist colleague in the form of scheduling the patient for an evaluation immediately, instead of making him wait for an available appointment. This would be a tangible communication to the patient that the physician is regretful about the oversight and that something is being done to make up for the error.

CALL FROM A NURSE

> *I'm the charge nurse this evening, and I want to ask you about something I learned on report. We have a patient, admitted yesterday, who is being treated with vancomycin for a serious cellulitis. Her nurse was very busy today; the next dose of vancomycin was delivered to the ward on time, but it was not actually administered until six hours after it was scheduled.*
>
> *The patient appears to be improving, and there doesn't seem to be any harm. Do we have to say anything to the patient or her family? If so, what should we say, and who should say it?*

DISCUSSION. This case raises several issues, such as what is the threshold for disclosure and who should be involved if disclosure occurs. In most workshops the group initially agrees that the patient should be told, but in further discussion it is often revealed that delays of this many hours are relatively common and that typically nothing is said to the patient. This leads into a discussion of whether our practices should change such that errors like this are routinely disclosed or, if not, where the threshold should be set. What if the delay in administration was only 2 hours, or 20 minutes, or 2 minutes? Presumably, at some point the delay is brief enough that disclosure is not likely to be necessary. Commonly, hospitals set a one-hour delay as the threshold for filing an incident report; perhaps this is also a reasonable threshold for disclosure as well.

The next question relates to the medical implications of the delay. Participants are generally in agreement that the charge nurse should inform the responsible physician, that a determination should be made as to whether this delay puts the patient at increased risk, and that steps should be taken to put the treatment back on course. From a medical perspective, a delay of this duration is unlikely to cause significant harm, but it is difficult to know for sure. In any event, the scheduling of the drug administration will need to be altered to adjust for the six-hour delay, and it may be necessary for some additional blood draws to be done to check drug levels. If the delay is not proactively disclosed, the patient might notice these changes in her care and ask about them, at which point it would be necessary either to lie (never a good option!) or to disclose the delay at that point, risking the appearance of an attempted cover-up.

If disclosure is to occur in this scenario, the next question is who should do it. Some participants recommend that the attending physician should have the conversation. Others feel this may inappropriately amplify the error and that the bedside nurse or charge nurse should explain to the patient what happened, apologize for the fact that the drug was administered late, explain that her physician has been notified, that adjustments to the dosing interval have been made, and that in all likelihood there will be no ill effects for the patient.

From the perspective of patient safety, this is an opportunity to make transparency more routine and to involve nurses directly in errors that occur as part of nursing practice. It is also an opportunity to involve the patient in monitoring her own care, in order to identify potential errors before they happen. If the patient in this scenario had been enlisted as a partner in patient safety and made aware of her medication schedule, she might have been able to remind the nurse that her next dose of medication was running late.

CALL FROM AN EMERGENCY DEPARTMENT (ED) PHYSICIAN

Earlier this evening we admitted a 19-year-old college student with signs of meningitis and septic shock. We intubated him, placed a central line, and resuscitated him with fluid and pressors. After he was stable on pressors, we took him to radiology for a head CT. We completed the CT, but moments after moving him from the scanner to his stretcher, we lost his blood pressure.

We quickly attempted resuscitation, but he never responded, and eventually we called the code. As we were preparing to take his body back to the ED, we realized that his CVL had become disconnected in the bed sheets and that none of his infusions or resuscitation medications had actually been administered. At this point, we were horrified to realize that the most likely reason he had coded was that he had not been receiving his pressors, and the most likely reason he did not respond to our attempt at resuscitation was because the medications were actually being administered into the bed sheets.

His CT scan showed massive cerebral edema and impending tentorial herniation, which the radiologist and I are convinced would have been lethal. We have just arrived back in the ED, and I am about to meet with his family and tell them that their son has died. Should I say anything to them about the problem with the CVL?

DISCUSSION. The premise of this case is that the error almost certainly did not change the ultimate outcome for the patient, since the patient had a rapidly fatal condition even before the error occurred. Even if the ultimate outcome is not in dispute, however, other aspects of the care might have been different. If he had not died in radiology, he likely would have been admitted to the ICU, giving his family a chance to spend some time with him before he died. If he had been diagnosed as brain-dead, it is possible his family might have gained some solace through the donation of his organs.

In all our workshops, this case provokes a fair amount of controversy. At times participants have been unanimous in the view that disclosure is not only not required but also would be cruel and inhumane. Given that the error almost certainly did not play a causative role in the young man's death, knowledge of this event could only be a source of pain for the family. It could also cause family members to falsely assume that the physicians would not have seen any reason to discuss the problem with the CVL if it was not a causative factor in the death.

In other workshops, participants have been equally adamant that disclosure is essential, while differing in terms of the reasons to disclose and the timing of the conversation. Some believe disclosure should occur simply because the family has a right to know the whole story, while others take a pragmatic approach, arguing that the family could learn the truth on their own at some point in the future, giving the impression of a cover-up. Some participants suggest that from a timing perspective there may be only one chance to disclose. The family may never return to the ED for a follow-up meeting, even if invited. At the same time, others argue that this is a family that is about to receive the sudden and unexpected news that their son, who was completely well until quite recently, is dead.

Disclosure in this instance may make the clinicians feel good about being transparent, but it may only further overwhelm the family at an already extremely traumatic time.

Regardless of the reasoning, the consensus generally emerges that if the clinicians choose not to disclose, they should document clearly the rationale behind their decision and why they believe the decision serves the best interests of the family. Whether their choice proves to be the best course or not, the contemporaneous documentation can convey a compassionate orientation toward the family and not be mistaken for trying to conceal important information.

CALL FROM A PSYCHIATRY ATTENDING

[Case contributed by Derri Shtasel, M.D.]

I have a young patient on the unit with a psychotic disorder. While we were in the middle of rounding, he began to pace rapidly and threaten other patients. I asked the nurse to offer him medication. (He has been refusing medication for the past two days and doesn't trust what I am "really" going to give him.)

I was surprised because he took the medication voluntarily and has been sleeping for the past three hours. The staff is pleased because a potentially volatile situation was safely and noncoercively defused. However, when I was reviewing his chart this morning, I realized that he received the wrong dose of the medication—actually twice as much as I'd intended. He's still paranoid but much calmer, has no physical side effects, and reports feeling much better than he had earlier. Do I need to tell him about this error?

DISCUSSION. Workshop participants are near unanimous in their recommendation not to disclose the error to this patient immediately, given the risk of exacerbating his psychiatric problems. They also acknowledge potential drawbacks to this decision, such as if the psychiatrist judges the increased amount of medicine to be a therapeutic dose, writes an order for the increase, and then must respond to the patient's request for an explanation for the increase.

Even if there is a decision not to disclose immediately, there is still the question of whether to disclose and when. Some suggest telling the patient's family about the error, but while this may satisfy the clinician's sense that she should tell someone, it may raise problems with confidentiality and may not address the clinician's ethical obligation to the patient. Participants are often uncertain about whether there is an obligation to disclose the error to the patient once he is no longer actively paranoid or whether, on balance, the therapeutic considerations justify a decision to waive disclosure altogether. In any case, there may be value in obtaining a second opinion from another psychiatrist and in documenting whatever decision is made, along with its rationale, in the medical record.

CALL FROM AN ICU ATTENDING

A 21-year-old was transferred to our ICU after three days of care in a community hospital ICU, where his condition had progressively worsened. On admission an hour ago he was in uncompensated septic shock, and he has just died.

In quickly reviewing his records from the referring hospital, I see that his admission KUB from three days ago had obvious free intraperitoneal air, likely indicating an intestinal perforation. There is no indication in the records that this finding was noted or recognized. I'm about to meet his parents. What should I say to them about why he died?

DISCUSSION. An age-old rule in medical etiquette is to never throw your colleagues "under the bus." Traditional practice would therefore be not to say anything to the family that would suggest an error on the part of the referring physicians and to assume that if the family is sufficiently motivated they will be able to find a lawyer, obtain the records, and discover the truth on their own. Workshop participants generally agree that this approach is outdated and unethical and that today we have positive obligations to inform family members of what we know.

Ideally and if circumstances permit, the physician should phone the referring hospital and inquire about the finding that was apparently missed. Perhaps it was not overlooked at all, and a good explanation will be given that can be passed on to the family. If this is not possible, the physician should inform the family of the facts, without attribution of blame, and suggest that the family return to the referring hospital for answers to their questions. This should always be followed by a phone call to the referring physicians to inform them of the findings and of what the family was told.

Most participants believe that this course of action would fulfill the ethical obligations of the clinicians. A minority have expressed the concern that this may not go far enough, since in their grief the family may not fully realize that their son's death may have been the result of a serious error and that the physician has an obligation to do at least some follow-up with the family to encourage them to follow through with the referring hospital and to obtain additional information.

This case also sometimes stimulates discussion about the role of radiologists and pathologists in disclosure of medical error. The American Medical Association Code of Ethics states that all physicians have obligations to their patients, even if this relationship is defined only through tests and procedures.[90] If a radiologist misreads an x-ray or a pathologist misinterprets a slide, do they have an obligation to personally disclose this error to the patient?[167] To our knowledge this is not current practice, but there are good reasons to think that it would be better for these specialists to be able to talk directly with the patients and families about the error rather than to have this information communicated through the primary clinicians.

CALL FROM A SURGEON

[Modified from Gallagher TH, Garbutt JM, Waterman AD, et al. Choosing your words carefully: how physicians would disclose harmful medical errors to patients. *Arch Intern Med.* August 14–28, 2006;166:1585.]

I just completed a cholecystectomy on one of my patients. I used this new laparoscopic device that our department just purchased. Everything was going well when one of our residents asked me a question. I turned off the device and looked in his direction to answer. When I turned back to the operative field, I saw that the device had burned a hole in the common bile duct. I was really surprised because the device I am used to using does not stay hot after it is turned off. We converted to an open procedure, and the remainder of the operation went well. I'm just about to go to the waiting room to speak with the patient's husband.

Do I have to tell him about the problems we had with the device? I would rather not, since I did get consent for both laparoscopic and open procedures. What if he asks me about why we could not perform the operation laparoscopically?

DISCUSSION. This case raises many issues not directly related to disclosure, such as the requirements for training before using a new device and whether patients should be informed when a physician is still learning about a technique or device that he or she intends to use.

The question of disclosure is not so much about whether to tell the husband but about what to say. For example, the surgeon could say, "Unfortunately we experienced the uncommon but well-known complication of burning the common bile duct, which required us to perform the cholecystectomy as an open procedure." This would not be lying, but it would not be telling the whole truth, either. However, minor distractions during surgery are not completely avoidable; this one just happened to occur at a particularly inopportune moment.

While there is no definitively correct way to disclose this event, perhaps the "Golden Rule" can serve as a guide for cases like this. Maybe the best advice is for the surgeon to honestly ask herself what she would like to be told if this incident were to happen to her or a close relative or friend.

CALL FROM AN INTERNIST

I just arrived at the hospital from home. One of my patients has died unexpectedly. She was a 42-year-old woman who was being treated for severe Crohn's disease. The residents told me she had an unexpected cardiac arrest at about 2 a.m. As they began the resuscitation, they sent labs from her CVL, which showed a serum potassium of 9 mEq/L.

During the code her PN solution was sent to the lab, and the potassium concentration was reported to be 10-fold higher than what was ordered. The resuscitation was not successful, and the house staff have already informed the family of her death but have said nothing about causation.

This is a family I have known for many years, and I feel terrible. When I meet with them in a few minutes, what should I say about why she died? Should I mention the potassium?

DISCUSSION. This is a situation in which it is very tempting to "connect the dots" and quickly assume that we understand what happened in this case. Everything makes sense—the high level of potassium in the PN, the high level of potassium in the blood, and the cardiac arrest. While this is certainly the most plausible explanation at the moment, and while it will likely turn out to be the correct explanation, the truth is that this conclusion is based on single lab determinations, obtained under chaotic conditions in the middle of the night, and not yet confirmed. Yet once a family has been told that their loved one died from incorrect preparation of the PN, it will be very difficult to backtrack with alternative explanations.

How much to disclose in this case depends a great deal on the relationship that the physician has with the family and how candid he thinks he can be with them without jeopardizing the relationship or their trust. While there are risks to offering a probable explanation too early, there are also risks to waiting so long that the family feels like they are having to drag the information out of the clinicians. Depending on the mix of factors, perhaps a middle-of-the-road explanation might work best here: "We are suspicious of some metabolic abnormalities as contributing to the cardiac arrest, we are actively investigating these now, and we will get back to you within the next couple of days with something more definitive."

CALL FROM A SURGEON

I'm up on the ward seeing a patient who is postop day #3 following abdominal surgery. She has developed a pretty nasty wound infection, which is slowly responding to treatment and getting better. The nurse has just pointed out to me that the patient missed a single dose of her routine perioperative antibiotics on postop day #1. She has confirmed with both the pharmacy and the nurse who had been working that day that the dose had not been given.

I really doubt that this had anything to do with why she developed a wound infection. So do I really need to tell her about the missing dose? If so, what should I say?

DISCUSSION. In our workshops, some have argued that since the value of prophylactic antibiotics in this setting has never been proven, there is no need to disclose. But of course if this surgeon really didn't think that they had any value, why did he order them in the first place?

The critical factors in this case seem to be the likelihood that the error played a causative role in the development of her wound infection and the magnitude of the potential harm to the patient. The greater each of these factors becomes, the greater is the obligation to disclose. Most likely, the missing dose played at most a minor role in the development of the wound infection, and most likely, the greatest harm would be a more prolonged recovery (although it is still possible that the infection could become a life-threatening issue). While these are judgment calls and a decision about whether to disclose could be defended either way, most of the participants in our workshops have felt that this case falls below the threshold requiring disclosure.

CALL FROM A PEDIATRICIAN

I just finished a meeting where I reviewed the death of a patient with her parents. She was an 8-year-old girl with Type 1 diabetes who was admitted with DKA. She came through the Emergency Department, met our clinical criteria for ward management, and was admitted to the general pediatric service. She was treated appropriately with our DKA protocol and seemed to be progressing well until late that evening, when her nurse found her to be barely arousable. A stat head CT was performed and showed cerebral edema. On review of her labs, her serum sodium had fallen from 138 to 135 to 132 over the first several hours. Usually serum sodium should rise with DKA treatment, and some think that a falling sodium is a "warning sign" for cerebral edema, but the data are not definitive. Despite transfer to the ICU and emergent management of her cerebral edema and intracranial hypertension, she developed cerebral herniation and died.

During the meeting her mother asked me, "Just tell me, doctor, was there anything that could have been done differently that might have saved her life." I didn't know what to say. Through the retrospectoscope, perhaps we should have picked up on the falling sodium and responded sooner. Even so, the outcome likely would have been the same. But if I answer honestly and tell the parents that, looking back, I might have done things a little differently, I'm sure they will think that I caused the death of their child and want to sue me. So I told them that nothing could have been done differently that might have saved her life. Did I do the right thing?

DISCUSSION. Although we often speak of honesty and transparency as ethical requirements, as with all ethical ideals they must be balanced against competing ethical considerations. If clinicians felt compelled to tell patients and families of every decision they considered in the treatment of every patient, our health care system would become paralyzed. Where is the balance between giving an honest and complete account of a patient's management and providing so much information and so many possibilities that the patient and family are left overwhelmed and confused?

A helpful analogy may be the conversations that we have with patients about their care in the absence of any concerns about error. When a physician tells a patient about a diagnosis, explains a prognosis, or prescribes a medication, the depth of the conversation is tailored to the context of the situation and the needs of the patient. For example, in prescribing a new medication, few—if any—physicians literally recite the long list of potential side effects that are listed in the *Physicians' Desk Reference* (*PDR*). Instead, most physicians mention only the most serious, the most common, or those that they think might be important to the patient given other issues of health or lifestyle; the physician then responds to the patient's questions or additional concerns. In other words, conversations between physicians and patients *always* fall short of including all the possible information that might be mentioned.

The problem with this analogy, of course, is that in routine conversations with patients physicians do not have any "skin in the game." The content of the conversation is dictated solely by the patient's desires and needs. In the context of adverse events, physicians are acutely aware that what they say might be used against them if the patient or family decides to pursue legal action. Given the competing interests that are at play, it can be very difficult to know where to draw the line between an honest and complete account of the patient's management and information that may be misleading or confusing.

Unfortunately, because of the personal risks involved, physicians are often inclined to err on the side of nondisclosure and to find reasons to justify the decision to themselves. Indeed, this is one of the key reasons that clinicians should seek the help of coaches before having these conversations, since the coach is in a better position to help with deciding what information is relevant and what is extraneous. In addition, if a physician's decision not to disclose is subsequently called into question, the physician involved is in a better position if he or she can say that an independent opinion was sought before making the decision.

TEN

Organizational Strategies for Improving Disclosure Practice

Improving communication in the aftermath of medical errors and adverse events will be successful only if it is part of a forward-looking organizational approach to promoting a culture of safety. Likewise, patient safety efforts, to be efficacious, must be part of a comprehensive strategy of organizational learning, which can be defined as "the social production of inter-subjective experiences and organizational rules, structures and relationships, leading to changed organizational behavior."[168] In this chapter, we explore specific strategies for learning and change that health care organizations can use to develop effective disclosure programs as part of a robust patient safety agenda.

Central to the process of organizational learning is the manner in which hospitals view, manage, and reflect on mistakes. Karl Weick, an organizational psychologist who has studied health care and other high-reliability organizations, suggests that when organizations become successful at reducing error and improving safety, it is because they learn to appreciate the "aesthetics of imperfection."[169] These organizations figure out how to learn from mistakes through an open process of collaboration and reflection among key stakeholders—patients, family members, health care professionals, staff, and administrators. High-reliability organizations invested in safety learn to examine traditional habits, assumptions, and patterns of thinking and to gauge progress not only with quantitative metrics but also by how well they are measuring up to the core relational values we have described in this book—transparency, respect, accountability, continuity, and kindness.

Optimal organizational learning depends on leadership at the highest levels but equally requires engagement and empowerment of staff at the levels of departments and frontline practice. Perhaps most important, it necessitates a heightened appreciation for a collaborative and relational form of learning that occurs in the context of appreciative and mutually respectful relationships. Within this framework, the knowledge and expertise of a high-functioning interdisciplinary team, for example, are understood to be a collective achievement, one that is greater than the sum of its individual parts.

Individuals and Systems

As health care organizations increasingly adopt more sophisticated ways of understanding and analyzing the systemic underpinnings of adverse events and medical errors, important questions arise about who is accountable for a given event and how accountability is best communicated to patients and families. When a serious event occurs, patients and families need to know that the clinicians most involved in their care are assuming responsibility for what has happened, and they need to hear from those clinicians directly. When an error is involved, they also need to receive an apology from those clinicians.

However, most errors that occur in health care organizations are not the fault of just one individual; rather, they reflect systemic, not-yet-addressed problems in the way health care is delivered. The patient safety movement reminds us that most medical errors are systemic and that a large percentage of them are preventable. Therefore, significant reductions in the rate of medical errors are tied more fundamentally to organizational priorities and how organizations learn than they are to the behaviors or proclivities of individual clinicians. In this respect, the health care organization itself, as much as the individual clinician, needs to be accountable to patients and families when errors occur.

These realities have implications for how errors should be explained to patients and families. The bottom line is that in any human enterprise like health care, when "human error" occurs, regardless of its cause, humans involved in that error must take responsibility and face the harmed party. In most cases, it is likely to be important to patients who have just suffered harm to know that the attending physician holds him- or herself responsible for the error because it occurred on his or her watch. At the same time, the communication must provide patients and families with an accurate understanding of the likely interdependent and systemic nature of the error. In addition, it requires that those health care professionals who are most directly involved in the event (including, for example, nurses, pharmacists, and physicians in training) be accountable and in communication with the patient and family. Resolving this tension—requiring individuals to express responsibility for the failures of systems and requiring individuals to communicate accountability while giving patients and families an accurate explanation of the complexity of the failure—can be a daunting challenge. Furthermore, although disclosure has traditionally been seen as the sole responsibility of the attending physician, it is becoming increasingly apparent that disclosure is the responsibility of all medical professionals, as well as the health care organization of which they are a part.

How organizations choose to address medical errors in this regard has significant impact not only on patients and families but on clinicians as well. When clinicians are involved in errors, whether they are the result of system inadequacies or not, they most often feel personally responsible. In situations in which unaddressed systems issues have caused the event, clinicians, too, may deserve a kind of organizational apology from their superiors; that is, they should receive a nonblaming message that alleviates the "shame and blame" dynamics that historically have surrounded these events and that acknowledges the learning and change that are yet to occur in health care organizations to eradicate preventable errors. The capacity of health care organizations to become increasingly transparent in this regard, to bring errors into the light of day without defensiveness, is critically important if they hope to address the internalized shame and secrecy that clinicians have historically had to live with in the aftermath of these events.[170] When adverse events and medical errors are widely discussed and clinicians understand that only a small minority of errors are the result of individual negligence, there is hope that the dynamics of shame and blame can give way to the kind of open and respectful learning that will lead to substantive improvements in patient safety.

Deciphering Mixed Messages

Despite the many potential benefits of disclosure, a substantial gap continues to persist between expectations for disclosure and current practice. This gap has persisted even though most health care organizations in the United States have adopted formal disclosure policies and many are implementing disclosure coaching programs. The persistence of this gap likely reflects the mixed messages that organizations continue to send regarding disclosure. These messages mirror the deep ambivalence that individual clinicians themselves experience related to this issue. For individual clinicians, the positive effects of transparency are often outweighed by a lack of confidence in their capacity to communicate effectively in these situations and by fears about negative consequences that may ensue.

On the organizational level, formal policies supporting disclosure are also frequently trumped by fears, such as harm to institutional reputation or damage to trust within the population of patients served. On a unit or departmental level, even when organizational leaders are voicing strong support for disclosure, residents may see their attending physicians pursuing a path of limited disclosure and conclude that this approach is the cultural norm within their specialty.

The potential benefits of a state-of-the-art workshop on improving disclosure can be quickly undone by overly cautious advice from a hospital risk manager when a real medical error occurs. These are prime examples of what has been called the "hidden curriculum" in health care, which, simply stated, is what health care professionals *do* in their day-to-day interactions with patients, families, and each other as opposed to what they say *should* be done in lectures and other formal settings.[171]

Improving transparency, in the form of open communication among patients, family members, and clinicians when an adverse event or medical error occurs, is difficult to accomplish in large part because it is wrapped up in historically established rules and dynamics within medical cultures that are inherently resistant to change. Those who are invested in organizational learning tied to disclosure need to appreciate the size of the task. Barriers to disclosure are deeply rooted in the human psyche as well as in conditioned fears about onerous legal consequences that might befall a physician who chooses to be honest. It is wise to be cognizant of the stubborn nature of these obstacles, not to become discouraged but rather to understand that the organizations most likely to succeed in these efforts will be those that adopt deliberate, multifaceted strategies designed to produce incremental but real changes over a period of time.

The 4-A Framework for Organizational Disclosure Strategies: Awareness, Accountability, Ability, and Action

The 4-A framework for organizational disclosure strategies, which consists of awareness, accountability, ability, and action, provides guidance to organizational leaders who are considering the kinds of policy-setting and learning activities that will be most conducive to improving disclosure within their institutions.[95] The core relational values, TRACK, as well as the practical disclosure guidelines offered in this book, can guide organizational learning in this area. Key to the learning that needs to happen, and to the change that needs to occur, is a commitment to strategies that include both "top down" and "bottom up" components. Table 8 summarizes some of the key points.

Promoting Awareness

The critical first component is to heighten awareness throughout the organization of the importance of disclosure. This includes educating clinicians about the gap between expectations for disclosure and current practice, as well as the consequences of this gap on patient trust and satisfaction, litigation, and patient safety. Since health care professionals and organizations generally consider themselves to be committed to the principle of transparency, they are likely to be unaware that disclosures often do not meet the hopes and expectations of patients and families. Without recognizing that there is a problem, health care organizations will understandably assign the issue of disclosure a lower place on the list of clinical and organizational practices that need improvement.

Awareness raising needs to take place at all levels of the organization, including frontline health care workers and extending all the way through the hospital trustees and CEO. A basic informational presentation about the importance of disclosure and data from across health care settings

TABLE 8. The 4-A Framework for Organizational Disclosure Strategies

Promoting awareness	Conduct grand rounds to review literature on the "disclosure gap" Conduct institutional assessment survey to measure attitudes of staff and leaders about disclosure Hold focus groups within the institution to assess local knowledge and needs Review actual disclosures within the institution and assess quality of disclosure Add disclosure as a templated discussion point for M&M conferences
Creating accountability	Track number of staff trained in disclosure skills Track percentage of events in which disclosure occurs Measure satisfaction of staff and patients with disclosure process Ensure that disclosure policies exist and are available Ensure availability of coaches around the clock
Developing disclosure ability	Provide broad-based education for all clinicians on the importance of disclosure Provide opportunities to build skills with simulation training Educate and support a cohort of clinicians to perform as coaches Provide for clinician support services, ideally making it a "normal" and routine aspect of follow-up
Turning ability into action	Engage institutional leadership in "top down" support of disclosure practices Provide opportunities to build and maintain skills with simulation training Link disclosure policies and procedures to other safety and quality initiatives Create mechanisms to provide a contact person for long-term communication with families after an error

Sources: Gallagher TH, Denham C, Leape L, Amori G, Levinson W. Disclosing unanticipated outcomes to patients: the art and practice. *J Patient Safety.* 2007;3:158–165. Denham C. Patient safety practices: leaders can turn barriers into accelerators. *J Patient Safety* 2005;1:41–55.

about the challenges of improving disclosure practice can be an effective first step in establishing awareness.

Another way to expand on organizational awareness is to conduct a local needs assessment to measure the attitudes of health care staff and leaders about disclosure. Published disclosure attitude surveys from the literature can be used for this purpose, and results for local cohorts can be compared with published norms.[99] An important part of this kind of needs assessment is to ask health care professionals how they might respond to specific disclosure scenarios. Using such scenarios will normally elicit greater variation in attitudes than more general questions about disclosure. Research indicating that physicians in different specialties have divergent disclosure attitudes can be used to engage various physician groups in the disclosure improvement process.[99,103,172] Surveying nonphysician health care providers is also key, since the consensus is growing that all members of the interdisciplinary team should be involved in the disclosure process.[173] Disclosure attitude questions can also be folded into safety culture surveys already being conducted by many organizations. Holding formal focus groups within the organization with different groups of health care professionals is an alternative strategy for assessing local needs.

One very effective strategy for enhancing awareness of the current state of disclosure within a health care organization is to share information and experiences regarding actual disclosures that have gone either well or poorly. At many organizations, a powerful driver of change with regard to patient safety is the occurrence of sentinel cases, assuming that the organization has the foresight and courage to cooperate with publicizing the case and to consciously use the event as a rallying cry for promoting change. On a less dramatic level, significant events can be openly reviewed within the organization as an explicit effort to learn about mistakes and how to approach them more productively. Many organizations use standard templates as a part of Morbidity and Mortality conferences to make sure that important safety variables are not overlooked. Adding items related to the disclosure process to the template—whether disclosure was appropriate, whether it occurred, and how it went—can be a relatively easy way to incorporate this topic into the routine review of adverse events.

A somewhat different strategy may be needed to promote awareness at the most senior levels of the organization. In many institutions, trustees and senior leadership only hear about the most serious adverse events and errors, many of which are so public and well known that disclosure is essentially inevitable. The trustees and leadership can mistakenly conclude from hearing about these cases that transparency regarding adverse events and errors is the norm, not recognizing that a disclosure performance gap may still exist, especially for less serious adverse events and errors. Regularly including considerations of disclosure as a standing agenda item at leadership meetings or providing them with the results of a local needs assessment can enhance senior leaders' awareness of the importance of improving the disclosure process. Senior leaders should be included in educational activities such as disclosure workshops. We have found the practice-based approach to learning described in earlier chapters—in which peers have the opportunity to enact, observe, and reflect on practice—to be most effective. For organizational leaders, this hands-on, realistic learning experience can be transformational and can help galvanize leadership support for directing necessary resources toward the creation of a comprehensive organizational support system for disclosure.

Throughout the awareness-raising process, organizations should be mindful, on the one hand, of ensuring interdisciplinary involvement at all levels and, on the other, of ensuring that physicians become and remain centrally involved. Physician involvement can be challenging in some institutions for several reasons, ranging from simple logistics such as getting busy clinicians to attend planning meetings to more challenging issues, such as where power and authority reside in relation to disclosure practices. Such barriers can lead organizations to consider diminishing the role of physicians in the learning and change process. Nonetheless, physician participation and buy-in needs to be an integral part of the process.

Creating Accountability

The second component in the 4-A framework is to establish clear accountability for the disclosure process. Organizations should delineate who is accountable for identifying and removing organizational barriers to disclosure and transparency, for making sure leadership and key staff are aware of predictable challenges and obstacles, and for securing the sufficient institutional resources to develop effective disclosure programs. A variety of process, structure, and outcome metrics can be developed to support such accountability. Process measures include the percentage of staff trained in disclosure, the frequency of events requiring disclosure for which disclosure was followed, and the satisfaction of staff with disclosure training and disclosure coaching services. Potential structure measures include verification that disclosure coaches are available around the clock, that pertinent disclosure policies exist and are available, that a process is in place to screen all unanticipated outcomes for consideration of disclosure, and that mechanisms exist to track whether and how disclosures occur. The presence of an internal disclosure reporting structure that includes senior administrative management and governance board leaders is another important structure measure. Over time, outcome measures related to disclosure can supplant the process and structure measures. These outcome measures include patients' trust in the integrity of the institution and the degree of satisfaction with disclosure among patients and family members who experience serious anticipated outcomes.

Disclosure can pose special challenges at hospitals that have private medical staffs, especially when a private physician has separate malpractice insurance coverage and disagreements occur between the physician and the organization about whether or how disclosure should take place. There is a natural tendency in these situations for the hospital and the private physician to implicitly or explicitly convey to the patient that primary responsibility for the event lies with the other party. While there is no magic bullet for resolving this issue, organizations with private medical staff should design policies and procedures with an eye toward promoting maximal collaboration with private physicians in relation to disclosure. Creating the perception in the mind of the patient that physicians or organizations are seeking to blame each other will only exacerbate the patient's distress and heighten the likelihood that a lawsuit will be filed. When possible, the hospital and private physician should approach the patient together, an approach that requires careful planning and consultation in advance of the actual disclosure conversation.

Developing Disclosure Ability

The third element in the 4-A framework is to enhance the ability of the organization to intervene effectively in the aftermath of adverse events and medical errors. The National Quality Forum safe practice on disclosure provides one potential model for implementing an organizational disclosure support system. Disclosure policies and procedures should be linked organizationally with other patient safety quality and improvement activities. These linkages will help to ensure that analysis of all unanticipated outcomes will include consideration of the disclosure itself and how it was carried out. It is also important that the reporting of a medical error to risk management become linked to other patient safety processes and that regular sharing of information about serious unanticipated outcomes and their disclosure occurs within leadership structures.

One key element of a disclosure support system is the identification and training of disclosure coaches or consultants as outlined previously in this book. Clinicians need to have around-the-clock access to this just-in-time guidance in order to effectively prepare for disclosures and to receive the support they need as clinicians. A vigorous disclosure support system also needs to provide learning activities focused on disclosure for all health care professionals in the organization. All health care workers need an understanding of basic disclosure concepts as well as the relevant organizational support resources and how they can be accessed.

A second key facet of a disclosure support system is developing and implementing formal mechanisms for supporting both patients and caregivers through the disclosure process. Effective intervention in the aftermath of a serious medical error normally extends for a considerable length of time. Patients and family members need a single point of contact within the organization, an individual who checks in with them proactively and whom they can call with questions as they arise. Often, organizations worry that such regular follow-up is unwise, reckoning that such contact may reopen wounds and remind patients of the trauma they suffered rather than facilitate their healing. However, when follow-up contact is compassionate and respectful, it can alleviate patients' experience of abandonment, validate their need to ask questions long after the event has occurred, and demonstrate to the patient and family the organization's commitment to efforts at repairing and restoring trust.

Support for the emotional impact of these events on health care workers is equally important. Historically, health care organizations have done a poor job of supporting health care professionals who have been involved in errors, and health care workers have been hesitant to reach out to those organizational support resources that do exist. Ensuring that the emotional responses of health care workers are normalized and addressed both in the immediate aftermath of a serious event and in the weeks and months that follow is a critical aspect of an effective disclosure program.

While disclosure has traditionally been conceived of as an individual physician talking with a patient, the growing consensus is in favor of an interprofessional approach, allowing all team members to offer input about what happened and contribute to the disclosure plan. A team approach also helps ensure that patients hear a consistent message about what happened. Productive interprofessional learning about adverse events and medical errors can be challenging, especially in the context of the power and authority gradients that shape relationships between physician and nonphysician team members. In light of this, disclosure coaches need to become skillful at creating a safe environment in which all voices can be heard.

The question of how many team members should participate in disclosure conversations with the patient and family is an area still under development. The advantages of having multiple team members participate include the ability to answer a wide range of patient questions about what happened, to make use of the different communication strengths of each team member, and to reinforce the message to the patient and family of how seriously the organization is taking the event. Potential disadvantages of too much team involvement include overwhelming the patient with multiple professionals and, in the absence of sufficient disclosure planning, conveying mixed messages about what has happened and what needs to happen next. Additional research is needed about how and in what circumstances team involvement is most effective.

A final key consideration in implementing disclosure policies and procedures is designing processes to ensure that the disclosures stay focused on the needs and preferences of each particular patient and family. Few circumstances stress our ability to deliver patient-centered care as much as the occurrence of a serious adverse event. Following such events, it is not uncommon for health care professionals and the organization itself to focus primarily on how the event and its disclosure affects them, potentially losing sight of the event's impact on the patient and family. These considerations can influence decisions regarding whether and how to carry out disclosures, as well as the actual disclosures themselves. Especially for disclosure of the most serious events, organizations should consider having safeguards to ensure that the patient perspective remains front and center during the period in which the decision is being made about whether disclosure is warranted. Formal consultation with the hospital ethics committee or patient advisory council is one strategy that can help to ensure ethically sound choices in these instances. Such consultation is especially warranted when considerations of nondisclosure are on the table, since such decisions, as discussed previously, should be required to meet a high ethical standard.

Turning Ability into Action

The final component of the 4-A framework is turning ability into action. If there is one lesson to be learned from the past decade of efforts by health care organizations and practitioners to improve disclosure of adverse events and errors to patients, it is how truly difficult it can be to translate the commitment to the principle of disclosure into practice. This difficulty in changing disclosure practices would come as little surprise to experts in organizational behavior, as current disclosure practices have deep roots in the culture of health care. Culture change with respect to any behavior can be difficult, but that difficulty is magnified when the behavior in question asks health care workers to have embarrassing, awkward, and challenging conversations with patients about adverse events and errors in the context of a litigious society. This slow pace of change regarding disclosure should prompt organizations to pay special attention to steps they can take to turn their awareness, accountability, and ability vis-à-vis disclosure into action.

One common obstacle that fledgling disclosure programs can experience involves unrealistic expectations among health care workers about likely outcomes of disclosure conversations. It is tempting for disclosure educators, when interacting with skeptical or scared clinicians, to emphasize the healing potential of effective disclosure conversations for both patients and providers and to remind clinicians of patients' strong desire that adverse events and errors be disclosed to them. While both of these messages are accurate, it is possible for clinicians to emerge from such programs believing that if they apply the recommended disclosure techniques, the conversation will end with the patient expressing his or her forgiveness of the clinician for what happened and thanking the clinician for being honest. This is an unrealistic and inappropriate expectation. Under normal circumstances, if the conversation goes well, it may end with the patient and family appreciating the clinician's openness but at the same time feeling a fair degree of anger, distress, and mistrust toward the clinician.

TABLE 9. Barriers to Disclosure and Potential Solutions

Barriers	Potential Solutions
Clinical Barriers	
Fear that disclosure will prompt litigation	Learn about relationship between disclosure and litigation
Concern that disclosure will not benefit the patient	Understand patients' preferences for disclosure, consequences of failed disclosure on patient-physician relationship
Lack of confidence in communication skills	Seek disclosure skills training, use disclosure coaches
Shame/embarrassment about error	Use institutional support resources
Institutional Barriers	
Concern that clinicians are not skilled in disclosure	Institute a disclosure support system, including training, coaching, and emotional support
Lack of awareness about deficiencies in disclosure practices	Measure quality of actual disclosures
Perception that disclosure is a risk management rather than a patient safety activity	Engage patients in safety and quality activities, including event analysis

Source: Gallagher TH. A 62-year-old woman with skin cancer who experienced wrong-site surgery: review of medical error. *JAMA*. 2009;302:669–677.

Clinicians can misread this as a failure. Ensuring that disclosure education and coaching instills realistic expectations among providers about the challenges of disclosure, and of the long time horizon around rebuilding trust with patients and families following a serious medical injury, can minimize the chances that clinicians will try disclosure once and then vow never to have a conversation like that again with a patient. Table 9 provides a summary of barriers to disclosure and potential solutions.

A fair criticism of many of the recommendations that we presented earlier in the book is that few of them can be adopted without significant organizational transformation. In this chapter we have tried to address some of these organizational challenges and how we might begin to meet them. In the final chapter we will look to the future and suggest some of the innovations that currently exist only on whiteboards and in e-mail memos but that are likely to be the areas of debate and progress over the next several years.

ELEVEN

Future Directions and Closing Thoughts

How clinicians communicate with patients and families in the aftermath of adverse events and medical errors has changed substantially over the past decade. At the same time, in many respects, competent and responsive disclosure practice is still at an early stage. Over the next several years, it is reasonable to expect that the pace of change will accelerate. In this chapter, we consider some potential areas for future development.

Linking Disclosure Quality and Safety Programs

Talking with patients and families about medical errors has long been seen primarily as a risk management issue. Progressive organizations are realizing, however, that improving practice in this domain is a key dimension of safe and high-quality health care. The integration of disclosure into institutional safety and quality programs will likely manifest itself in a variety of ways. For example, these programs at many institutions have evolved to the point where "dashboards" have been developed so that clinicians can see at a moment's notice which of their patients are currently out of compliance with key quality guidelines, such as preventive screening or adequate glucose control. A similar approach is likely to develop with regard to disclosure, which would require developing systems that monitor when a event has taken place that requires disclosure, track whether a disclosure conversation has occurred, and report the patient's assessment of the quality of that conversation. Systems such as these will enable health care organizations to intervene in real time when disclosures do not occur or do not go well.

Improved disclosure practice, occurring at the "sharp end" of health care organizations, will also increasingly become a driver of quality improvement efforts. For example, since patients and family members often witness adverse events and medical errors, they have a unique perspective and may have key information that can be gleaned from frank and respectful disclosure conversations. Information learned from the patient can be fed into the quality improvement process, enhancing the effectiveness of the analysis and strengthening plans for preventing recurrences. Patients can also be included in root cause analysis procedures so that they can convey their perspective directly to safety experts about what took place. Integrating patients into quality and safety activities depends on openly and empathically disclosing the event to patients in the first place. Equally important, it requires a shift in the extent to which the knowledge of patients and family members is valued and respected within health care organizations. It also requires the courage, on the part of health care leaders, to heed the consistent message of the patient safety movement: "Nothing about us, without us."

Improved disclosure practice is an essential ingredient within health care organizations committed to transparency. Enacting the value of transparency requires organizations to recognize the important parallel between, on the one hand, clinicians being open with patients and family members about adverse events and, on the other, clinicians being open within their institutions about the *occurrence* of those events. Indeed, some countries, such as the United Kingdom, have abandoned the term "disclosure" in favor of the broader concept of "being open." Many organizations are beginning to include disclosure practices when measuring institutional safety culture, and disclosure initiatives are being integrated into the broader emphasis on promoting a "just culture" in health care.

When optimal communication with patients and families in the aftermath of adverse events and medical errors is openly advocated as an institutional priority and responsibility, rather than as the sole province of the attending physician, improved disclosure practice will become an expectation throughout health care systems, including as part of credentialing and privileging processes. Holding health care professionals accountable in these ways for adhering to organizational disclosure policies will send a powerful message that the expectation of improved practice in this domain of patient care is here to stay.

Rebuilding Trust in Ruptured Relationships

Living up to the core relational values we have discussed in this book—transparency, respect, accountability, continuity and kindness—represents the ultimate challenge to health care organizations invested in transforming themselves as we enter the second decade of the twenty-first century. Adverse events and medical errors occur in a network of human relationships, and the values at the core of these relationships are shaken and called into question at the time of a serious event. Often, relationships are strained at every level—between clinicians and patients, between clinicians and clinicians, and between clinicians and administrators. When relationships are ruptured, it is critical that organizations do their utmost to live up to these values, for the sake of patients and families who have been harmed, for the sake of the clinicians involved, and for the sake of the institution as a whole. The occurrence of a serious medical error constitutes an important crossroads for any health care organization, an ethical moment when, in words borrowed from *Death of a Salesman*, "attention must be paid."

At the time of such events, the foremost ethical demand is to respond competently and compassionately to the needs of the patient and family. The natural impulses of clinicians at these times can be self-protective in ways that can distract from providing good patient-centered care. The art of communicating well with patients and families at these difficult times is in its infancy. While the existing literature highlights patients' desire for disclosure of adverse events and errors, little is known about the range and variation of patients' needs at these times.

Although the first priority should always be responding to the needs of patients and families, the immediate next priority must be to provide support, guidance, and positive learning experiences for the clinicians involved. Setting up support systems and making clinicians aware of their availability is an important step. However, the barriers to accessing such support are substantial, embedded as they are in the fabric of medical culture. If a physician, for example, operates with the assumption that good doctors do not make mistakes, the occurrence of a medical error, even if it is one that could happen to any clinician, is understandably viewed as a personal failure. Moreover, seeking help for such a transgression is likely to be seen as a further sign of weakness. It is therefore vital, in developing organizational strategies for supporting clinicians in these contexts, to normalize the occurrence of medical error as part of a comprehensive patient safety strategy within which serious errors, however unfortunate, are seen as positive opportunities for learning. All clinicians involved in an adverse event can be part of a "checking-in" process by trusted peers, one that occurs over time and adjusts the level and nature of support to the needs and coping styles of each clinician. These kinds of systems are largely undeveloped thus far, but they are a vital component of a robust and significant organizational strategy for addressing medical error.

Promoting Collaborative Disclosure Conversations and Offers of Compensation to Patients in All Health Care Settings

As discussed previously, many large self-insured organizations such as the University of Michigan, the University of Illinois at Chicago, and Stanford University have reported success when coupling open disclosure with early offers of compensation. Private malpractice insurers including COPIC, ProMutual, and West Virginia Mutual have also instituted disclosure and compensation programs, though on a more limited scale. What has yet to emerge, however, are models of effective collaborative approaches to disclosure and offers of compensation in settings where the physician and health care institution do not share a malpractice insurer. At present, when a significant error occurs at a health care organization with a private medical staff, the natural tendency is for the respective malpractice insurers to direct the maximal blame for the events, with the associated financial responsibility, to the opposing party. Collaboration between different malpractice insurers on disclosure and compensation strategies has also been limited by challenges inherent in sharing confidential, peer-reviewed and -protected event analysis and information.

Considerable analysis and research are needed to understand how disclosure and compensation models that have succeeded in self-insured settings can be applied to the far larger number of settings in which care is delivered. Clearly, such collaborative attempts at disclosure and compensation will be more effective for some types of medical injuries than for others. Private malpractice insurers and health care institutions should seek out the opportunity for partnerships with regard to disclosure and compensation, perhaps by first identifying a subset of events in which collaboration would be most feasible. In states where information shared with patients during settlement negotiations is protected from discovery, such collaboration between a private insurer and a health care organization might be framed under the broader settlement umbrella to benefit from similar protection from discoverability.

Reforming the National Practitioner Data Bank

The central idea underlying the National Practitioner Data Bank (NPDB), namely, the need for a national system for tracking providers whose competence is in question, makes sense. Unfortunately, the NPDB has been implemented in ways that can have an inhibiting effect on disclosure, especially when the medical error is one that is going to be linked to compensation. Practitioners need to be reported to the NPDB when a payment is made on their behalf in response to a written demand from a patient, among other reporting requirements. Yet in many instances, payments made to patients following adverse events or errors do not necessarily reflect substandard care by an individual provider but rather a series of system failures. In addition, some large self-insured entities have chosen to settle all claims on behalf of the organization instead of naming individual providers and therefore do not report even large payments made to patients to the NPDB. Nonetheless, when physicians *are* reported to the data bank, it makes the subsequent processes of renewing their medical license or obtaining hospital privileges more complex. Reforming the data bank reporting procedure to focus more on measures of competence rather than the occurrence of payouts could mitigate concerns about the data bank being a barrier to the disclosure process.

New Educational Models

There is much to be learned about effective strategies for educating health care professionals about disclosure. In this book, we have described our own practice-based approach to learning that we have found to be promising. Many health care institutions have created sophisticated and detailed disclosure policies and procedures, which is an important first step. The development of just-in-time tools such as e-learning tutorials can support clinicians when disclosing minor and moderate errors, situations in which it may not be necessary to activate more formal coaching interventions.

An especially challenging task is how to provide health care professionals in training with the appropriate skills in disclosure. At most organizations, the attending physician will continue to be the person who is primarily responsible for disclosures. This expectation, however, can result in new physicians, not to mention nurses and other health care professionals, entering practice with no formal training or exposure to communicating with patients and families at these times. Learning opportunities for medical students, residents, nursing students, and others should include didactic background material as well as the opportunity to practice disclosures in role-play enactments. In addition, clinicians in training can learn important skills by accompanying more senior colleagues, when appropriate, during disclosure conversations. Effective educational strategies will also address the impact of the hidden curriculum, identifying those mixed messages that trainees receive about disclosure. Learning about disclosure may also need to be customized by specialty and discipline, given the different ways in which health care professionals approach the process.

Filling the Research Gap

Research supporting improved disclosure practice has grown rapidly over the past few years, but important knowledge gaps persist. Research is needed to better understand the unique needs and preferences of patients and families based on differences in gender, race, class, and ethnicity. A thoughtful, ethical approach to patients and families based on their unique characteristics could improve disclosure practice overall, as well as help to identify those circumstances in which nondisclosure may be warranted. As our understanding of effective disclosure strategies continues to increase, disclosure policies and procedures will become more firmly evidence based.

Perhaps most important, the synergistic importance of linking disclosure policies and programs with those in patient safety and quality improvement should not be underestimated, particularly when disclosure is combined with structures that facilitate early compensation for certain types of injury. The organizational challenges to these types of innovation can be daunting, but the payoff—in terms of improved quality and safety of care, the satisfaction of patients and families with their experience of involvement and partnership with clinicians, and the reduced levels of stress and burnout among clinicians—makes these challenges well worth the effort. Future research can help to determine the best practice models for achieving integration within this complex array of interactions.

This vision of future directions brings the themes of this book full circle. We began by identifying the need for better communication in the aftermath of adverse events and medical errors. We have explored the ways in which clinicians can improve their ability to have these conversations at the bedside with patients and families and the crucial importance of recognizing the emotional needs of clinicians at these difficult times. We have also acknowledged that these efforts cannot, in the long run, succeed without a determined commitment on the part of health care leaders to enact core relational values of transparency, respect, accountability, continuity, and kindness and to support organizational learning that will lead to change.

The capacity of health care organizations to become more truly transparent and to appreciate the "aesthetic of imperfection" will result not only in improved disclosure practice but also in a new generation of clinicians who are naturally invested in speaking up when error occurs, in the interest of everyone's learning. Organizational commitment to improved disclosure practice, integrated within a comprehensive program of patient safety, will result in fewer and less serious errors, creating less need to have disclosure conversations with patients and families in the first place. Implementing this vision in the years ahead will be challenging, for reasons that have been outlined in this book. Ultimately, however, it is well worth the effort because it is the right thing to do.

Appendix

Practical Guidelines for Disclosure

First Priorities

- Ensure that the clinical team stays fully attentive to the medical needs of the patient.
- Ensure that key individuals are notified and involved as soon as possible, including the attending physician and the hospital risk manager.
- Contact a designated "coach" and make arrangements for a meeting to plan disclosure.
- If the adverse event involved medical equipment or devices, ensure that these have been sequestered for later investigation.

Preparation for the Disclosure Conversation

- Approach clinicians collaboratively and use the ask-tell-ask method.
- Gather information about the eent from all the clinicians involved.
- Determine whether the adverse event meets the threshold requiring disclosure to the patient or family.
- Remind the team that this conversation is for the benefit of the patient and family and that the needs of clinicians will be addressed separately.
- Determine which clinicians should be present for the initial conversation.
- Assess who should be present for support of the patient and family.
- Decide who should lead the conversation.
- Agree on the core information that will be communicated.
- Determine an optimal time and setting for the conversation.
- Decide who will take primary responsibility for following up, so that this can be communicated unambiguously to the family.
- Discuss with the team how the patient's culture, health literacy, disabilities, and level of sedation may impact the conversation.

The Conversation with the Patient and Family

- Bring your own caring and humanness to the conversation.
- Remember the core relational values that can help to rebuild relationships when trust has been ruptured.
- Apply the "Golden Rule": What would you want to be told if you were the patient?
- Convey compassion and empathy for the patient's and family's suffering.
- Set the agenda for the meeting.
- Communicate collaboratively by using the ask-tell-ask method.
- Clearly state the facts as they are known at the present.
- Consider whether this is one of the rare circumstances in which disclosure of the facts may not be of immediate benefit to the patient/family.
- Convey caring always, and apologize when appropriate.
- Explain what is being done to care for the patient and the plan for care going forward.
- Assess whether the existing clinical relationships can be maintained or whether care needs to be transitioned to alternative providers.
- Assure the patient/family that the event will be thoroughly investigated and that all facts will be communicated as they become known.
- Acknowledge that questions about financial compensation are appropriate and legitimate and that they will be addressed by others with the qualifications and authority to do so.
- Offer support services—chaplains, social workers, patient advocates.
- Remember that disclosure may not be greeted with thanks or forgiveness.

Documentation and Follow-up

- Debrief the event, whenever possible, with a postconversation huddle.
- Assess the emotional and psychological needs of the clinicians involved and ensure follow-up for clinicians impacted by the event.
- Document the conversation in the medical record.
- Do not document the coaching intervention in the medical record.

Annotated Bibliography of Key Works

Background and Incidence of Medical Error

Brennan TA, Leape LL, Laird NM, et al. Incidence of adverse events and negligence in hospitalized patients: results of the Harvard Medical Practice Study I. *N Engl J Med.* 1991;324:370–376.

The Harvard Medical Practice Study (HMPS) was designed to obtain empirical data about adverse events, negligence, and malpractice claims. The study included a review of a large, randomized sample of medical records of patients discharged from nonpsychiatric hospitals in New York in 1984. This review reveals a high incidence of adverse events and negligence. Specifically, the authors estimate a statewide rate of adverse events among hospitalized patients of 3.7 percent (or 98,609 events) and a rate of adverse events caused by negligence of 1 percent (or 27,179). The methodology and findings of the HMPS proved influential in future research and policy discussions.

Thomas EJ, Studdert DM, Burstin HR, et al. Incidence and types of adverse events and negligent care in Utah and Colorado. *Med Care.* 2000;38:261–271.

Using methods similar to the HMPS and reviewing the records of 15,000 patients discharged from nonpsychiatric hospitals in Utah and Colorado in 1992, Thomas and colleagues arrive at relatively similar results. Although the estimates for the occurrence of adverse events (2.9%) and the percentage of those caused by negligence (27.5 in Colorado and 32.6 in Utah) are slightly lower, the authors conclude that iatrogenic injuries remain a significant problem.

Institute of Medicine [U.S.]. Committee on Quality of Health Care in America. *To Err Is Human: Building a Safer Health System.* Washington, DC: National Academy Press; 2000.

This landmark report, presenting evidence of the high frequency and cost of medical error, provided the impetus for the growth of the patient safety movement of the twenty-first century. The report examines the nature of error, concluding that much error in medicine is systems based and must be addressed on a systemwide basis. The report promotes error reporting and protection of information voluntarily reported. It offers numerous specific recommendations for creating safer systems in health care. This report was followed by several other influential IOM reports on patient safety.

Reason JT. *Human Error.* Cambridge, England: Cambridge University Press; 1990.

Reason's classic text on human error has three major subdivisions: an introduction to the concepts and research regarding human error; a presentation of basic error mechanisms; and a review of the consequences of human error. Reason's detailed study and rich analysis inform much of the later work on medical error.

Disclosure: General Overview

Banja JD. *Medical Errors and Medical Narcissism.* Sudbury, MA: Jones and Bartlett Publishers; 2004.

Banja focuses on responses of health care professionals/organizations to error and the degree of—and reasons for—nondisclosure. He acknowledges that fear of litigation has contributed to nondisclosure but also introduces, as another factor, a type of narcissism that may be fostered by medical training and practice. Banja also explores the psychological and moral characteristics of forgiveness and its place in the aftermath of harmful error. He suggests three kinds of support that would contribute to increased disclosure: a structured teaching curriculum (including role-modeling); the bolstering of the moral environment within which clinicians practice; and tort reform. Finally, he examines the nature and role of empathy in professional-patient interactions, giving examples of empathic techniques and responses. He provides suggestions for, and examples of, the content and process of disclosure.

Baylis F. Errors in medicine: nurturing truthfulness. *J Clin Ethics* 1997;8:336–340.

In this early article, Baylis examines and counters common justifications for not disclosing (or only partially disclosing) medical error: uncertainty about whether an error has occurred; the belief that disclosure only increases patients' suffering; and fear of litigation. She posits an even more encompassing reason: the culture of medicine, which accepts, and may even encourage, nondisclosure. Baylis recommends that the profession encourage disclosure by developing a more open, supportive environment among clinicians; em-

phasizing truthfulness as the foundation of the patient-physician relationship; working to support appropriate tort reform; and acknowledging that medical professionals (like other humans) are fallible.

Berlinger N. *After Harm: Medical Error and the Ethics of Forgiveness.* Baltimore, MD: Johns Hopkins University Press; 2005.

Berlinger's work examines the emotional and psychological aftermath of medical harm using concepts derived from religious tradition. (The author offers evidence that such concepts have become part of our secular culture.) Her focus is on how the patient, family, and physician experience the medical harm and on the subsequent steps that occur, from disclosure to apology to repentance and forgiveness. This book draws on major works in narrative ethics, Christian ethics, feminist ethics, legal scholarship, philosophy, and sociology. Building on her theoretical analysis, the author presents concrete recommendations for acting ethically in the face of medical error.

Gallagher TH, Bell SK, Smith KM, Mello MM, McDonald TB. Disclosing harmful medical errors to patients: tackling three tough cases. *Chest* 2009;136: 897–903.

Gallagher and colleagues posit that the discrepancy between the principle of disclosure of medical error and actual practice (which often falls short of full disclosure) stems at least in part from complexities and challenges not yet fully understood or resolved. The authors illustrate this point using three "hard" cases that contain uncertainties, gray areas, and mixed motives. In the discussion of each case, the authors acknowledge the arguments that might initially seem to support non- (or limited) disclosure. However, they demonstrate that a careful scrutiny of the facts, reasoning, and motivations leads to the conclusion that the patient/family should be provided with all "material" information (a term discussed by the authors). It is helpful that in each case the authors state their "bottom line" in regard to disclosure.

Gallagher TH, Studdert D, Levinson W. Disclosing harmful medical errors to patients. *N Engl J Med.* 2007;356:2713–2719.

This article provides an update on the practice of disclosure of medical error to patients. It offers a succinct summary of the prevalence of medical error, the history and current status of the practice of disclosure, regulatory responses in the United States as well as in several other countries, guidance from accrediting agencies (with special attention to the National Quality Forum safe practices guidelines), legal issues and developments, and important ongoing disclosure programs. The authors note that until more research results are available, disclosure standards will probably remain advisory; nonetheless, they predict that within a decade, disclosure will be the norm.

Mazor KM, Simon SR, Gurwitz JH. Communicating with patients about medical errors: a review of the literature. *Arch Intern Med.* 2004;164:1690–1697.

Mazor and colleagues point out the results, methods, strengths, and weaknesses of the studies available at the time. In particular, they identify 17 articles reporting results of key empirical studies on disclosure of preventable medical errors to patients/families (out of a total of 833 works). Based on their review, the authors posit three stages of disclosure. Studies on stage one, the disclosure decision, show that a large majority of patients want to be told about medical error. Physicians also generally support disclosure, particularly when harm occurs; nonetheless, in responding to specific scenarios and questions, they report a fairly high percentage of cases in which they would not disclose. (The authors report far fewer studies on the next two stages, process and consequences of disclosure and recommend further areas for research.)

American Society for Healthcare Risk Management of the American Hospital Association. Disclosure of unanticipated events: the next step in better communications with patients [first of three parts]. May 2003. www.ashrm.org/ashrm/resources/monograph.html. Accessed June 12, 2008.

This monograph offers a brief historical perspective on disclosure, highlighting the development of Patient Safety Standards by the Joint Commission on the Accreditation of Healthcare Organizations, which require that patients be informed of adverse outcomes of care. While acknowledging that the standards do not provide detailed guidance for disclosure, the monograph stresses that providers should be less concerned about the exact parameters of what "must" be disclosed and more concerned about creating an environment of open communication designed to foster patient safety. The monograph identifies key psychological and legal barriers to disclosure. It also presents several models for managing disclosure, along with examples of specific disclosure situations. ASHRM produced several subsequent, useful monographs on disclosure.

Rubin SB, Zoloth L, eds. *Margin of Error: The Ethics of Mistakes in the Practice of Medicine.* Hagerstown, MD: University Publishing Group; 2000.

Rubin and Zoloth have edited a rich collection of essays by leaders in the field of medical ethics. Articles in the first section of the collection focus on conceptual aspects of medical error; those in the second section discuss errors in the practice of medicine; and those in the third section explore error in the context of ethics consultation.

Smith ML, Forster HP. Morally managing medical mistakes. *Cam Quarterly of Healthcare Ethics.* 2000;9:36–53.

The authors explore key questions surrounding medical error: what is an error; why do errors occur; what happens to professionals and patients when they do; should they be disclosed; if so, why and to whom. They describe the context in which errors occur, including the medical culture of perfectionism, the tensions within the physician-patient relationship, and the medical malpractice system. Applying ethical theory (including rights-based and duty-based theories, virtue ethics, and consequentialism), they conclude that disclosure should become standard practice, with limited exceptions. They note that medicine can learn from other industries that have tackled the problem of human error. Finally, the authors propose action items for improving the handling of medical error, including training for medical and allied health students, continuing education programs for professionals, emphasis on quality improvement strategies, establishment of institutional policies and guidelines, revision of professional codes of ethics, incorporation of error disclosure into the concept of informed consent, modification of malpractice policies and strategies, and tort reform.

Wojcieszak D, Saxon JW, Finkelstein, MM. *SorryWorks! Disclosure, Apology, and Relationships Prevent Medical Malpractice Claims.* Bloomington, IN: AuthorHouse; 2007.

The authors are members of the SorryWorks! Coalition, which encourages expressions of empathy in the aftermath of medical error. This text includes chapters on how to implement a Sorry Works! Program, how and why such a program works, and how to apologize. Communications after an adverse event should almost always include an expression of empathy—"I'm sorry." An acceptance of responsibility and an apology are appropriate in a small proportion of the cases, when due diligence reveals that an error has occurred.

Wu AW, Cavanaugh TA, McPhee SJ, Lo B, Micco GP. To tell the truth: ethical and practical issues in disclosing medical mistakes to patients. *J Gen Intern Med.* 1997;12:770–775.

Writing prior to the IOM report, Wu and his colleagues note that medical errors are "common" but physician disclosure of such errors is not. They conclude that such disclosure is ethically obligatory if the error is made by the physician (not a systems error) and causes significant harm that is likely to be remediable, mitigable, or compensable. They base their argument on ethical theories such as consequentialism, deontology, the fiduciary nature of the physician-patient relationship, and the principles of biomedical ethics. The authors offer suggestions on practical issues (such as when and how an error should be disclosed, and by whom). They suggest that the conversation with the patient include a statement by the physician that he or she made an error; an explanation of the course of events (including the nature of the mistake and consequences); information as to corrective action taken; an expression of personal regret; an apology; and mitigation of financial costs, as appropriate. The authors recognize and respond to the pragmatic reasons that physicians might not want to disclose, and they encourage the development of guidelines for disclosure, support for physicians, and system changes.

Disclosure, Risk Management, and Liability

Kachalia A, Shojania KG, Hofer TP, Piotrowski M, Saint, S. Does full disclosure of medical errors affect malpractice liability? the jury is still out. *Joint Comm J Qual Saf.* 2003; 29:503–511.

While the fear of liability has been identified as an important barrier to disclosure of medical errors, these authors report that an extensive review of published medical and legal literature reveals little empirical data showing the effect of disclosure on malpractice risk. (They found one published study that revealed that malpractice liability decreased after implementation of a policy of disclosure at the VA Medical Center in Lexington, Kentucky, but concluded that the results are hard to generalize given the unique nature of a federal hospital system.) Thus, while disclosure is supported by ethical, safety, and justice concerns, further study is necessary to determine whether disclosure increases malpractice risk.

Studdert DM, Mello MM, Gawande AA, Brennan TA, Wang YC. Disclosure of medical injury to patients: an improbable risk management strategy. *Health Aff* (Millwood). 2007; 26:215–226.

Studdert and colleagues hypothesize that disclosure of medical error will not reduce malpractice claims; instead, any reduction achieved through a policy of disclosure will be countered or negated by the increase prompted by such disclosure. They test this hypothesis by performing Monte Carlo simulations on a model based on existing epidemiological data regarding medical injuries and malpractice claims, plus expert opinion regarding likely patient response to disclosure. Analyzing the results, the authors conclude that while disclosure is the right thing to do, it is highly likely to result in an increase in amount and cost of litigation. Although additional empirical data are necessary to test the hypothesis further, the results of the study challenge the assumption that disclosure can be justified by reduction in malpractice claims and costs.

Disclosure and Views of Patients and Providers

Duclos CW, Eichler M, Taylor L, et al. Patient perspectives of patient-provider communication after adverse events. *Int J Qual Health Care.* 2005;17:479–486. *This study examines the effect of patient-provider communications in situations involving actual adverse medical events. Subjects were recruited from a pool of patients identified by COPIC, Inc., a physician malpractice insurer in Colorado, as part of an early intervention program. In each case, the adverse event had required extensive medical follow-up. In focus groups conducted with these patients and several family members, all participants reported physical trauma, and many reported emotional trauma as well (although those who reported good communications with their providers reported less). Many patients/families also experienced financial distress because of the cost of follow-up care. Patients also revealed that they were worried about what had happened and what would happen next. They became angry if they had to fight to get information. (Most patients were angrier about how they were treated than about the event itself.) All patients who indicated that the communication process had not gone well reported no continuing relationship with the provider. Patients who reported good communication were more likely to continue the relationship and more likely to perceive the event as a "mistake" rather than incompetence. The study also noted patient/family sensitivity to the tone of conversations (i.e., whether providers seemed to be acting in fear of a lawsuit, or attempting to "cover up").*

Fein SP, Hilborne LH, Spiritus EM, et al. The many faces of error disclosure: a common set of elements and a definition. *J Gen Intern Med.* 2007;22:755–761. *Fein and colleagues conducted focus groups for clinicians and administrators at academic medical centers that had adopted a policy of disclosing medical error to patients. Participants were encouraged to express their views about disclosure of error generally and to respond to a specific hypothetical. Most participants said they would report a medical error to a patient. However, some of the disclosures described by the participants (either in connection with actual cases or in response to the hypothetical) did not meet the authors' definition of "full disclosure." (The six elements of "full disclosure" were garnered from the qualitative analysis.) Disclosures were often "partial," a category that the authors further divided into three subcategories: (1) "connect the dots" (failing to link the error and the effect), (2) "mislead" (implying that error was part of the natural condition or expected complication of treatment) or (3) "defer" (suggesting other possibilities when the error is known). Responses considered "partial disclosure" or nondisclosure accounted for the majority of all the disclosures in the study. Based on the study, the authors propose a definition of "disclosure" that will assist clinicians in achieving full disclosure.*

Gallagher TH, Garbutt JM, Waterman AD, et al. Choosing your words carefully: how physicians would disclose harmful medical errors to patients. *Arch Intern Med.* 2006; 166:1585–1593.

The authors surveyed 2,637 U.S. and Canadian physicians about whether and how they would disclose information after one of four hypothetical errors. The results reinforced the findings in prior studies that there is a gap between what patients seem to want and what physicians provide after medical error. For example, despite past studies indicating that patients desire accountability, apology, and information (including what will be done to prevent future error), physicians in the study tended not to use the word "error"; not to frame a specific apology; and not to provide information about actions that would be taken to prevent a similar error. Overall, physicians were more apt to disclose an error if it was obvious, and not to disclose if it seemed that patients would not otherwise know about it. Based on their work, the authors counsel the development of disclosure standards and training.

Gallagher TH, Waterman AD, Ebers AG, Fraser VJ, Levinson W. Patients' and physicians' attitudes regarding the disclosure of medical errors. *JAMA.* 2003; 289:1001–1007.

The authors report on a study in which 13 focus groups (composed of patients or physicians or both) were presented with hypothetical situations involving medical error. A qualitative analysis of the transcripts of the sessions reveals a number of important differences in the attitudes of patients and physicians, including: (1) patients conceived of medical errors more broadly than physicians; (2) patients wanted to be told about any error that caused them harm, whereas physicians, while generally agreeing, described situations in which they would not disclose; (3) patients wanted full disclosure (including what happened, how their health would be affected, why it happened, what would be done to fix it and prevent future errors) and an apology, but some physicians were more cautious about what they would disclose (many noting the fear of litigation and the need to avoid language suggesting liability). In regard to "near misses," patient preferences regarding disclosure were mixed, while physicians generally opposed disclosure. Both patients and physicians reported that errors would cause them emotional distress. The article includes recommendations for how to respond to medical error, including minimum disclosure requirements and better institutional support for the emotional needs of the practitioner.

Gibson R, Singh JP. *Wall of Silence: The Untold Story of the Medical Mistakes That Kill and Injure Millions of Americans.* Washington, DC: LifeLine Press; 2003.

This book presents a series of dramatic patient/family stories illustrating the consequences of medical error. In most cases, patients or families report not receiving full information about what happened or an acknowledgment of responsibility or an expression of sorrow. While focusing on personal stories (including that of the authors), the book also includes a brief summary of the IOM report; a discussion of the so-called wall of silence (the professional practice of not disclosing error to outsiders); and brief discussions of what constitutes "medical error," reasons for such errors, grassroots resources for patients/families, and suggestions for working toward reducing future errors.

Hilfiker D. *Healing the Wounds: A Physician Looks at His Works.* New York: Pantheon Press; 1985.

Dr. Hilfiker's classic work is an account of the pressures of practicing medicine—with its inherent uncertainties, the inevitability of mistake, and the inadequacy of training and support for physicians facing such pressures. His open acknowledgment of his own errors, and the emotional consequences, encouraged a more open discussion among clinicians of their own, similar experiences.

Mazor KM, Simon SR, Yood RA, et al. Health plan members' views about disclosure of medical errors. *Ann Intern Med.* 2004;140:409–418.

In this study, surveys were sent to 1,500 representative members of a large health plan (response rate 66%). The surveys presented vignettes that varied as to type of error, clinical outcome, and extent of disclosure. In general, full disclosure increased patient satisfaction and positive emotional response and decreased the likelihood the patient would change physicians. Full disclosure did not, however, ensure a positive response; patients were also influenced by the specifics of the error and severity of the outcome. In only one vignette did disclosure reduce the likelihood of legal action. Member responses to general questions confirmed that patients want a detailed explanation of a medical error, a sincere apology, and assurance that steps will be taken to avoid recurrence.

Shannon SE, Foglia MB, Hardy M, Gallagher TH. Disclosing errors to patients: perspectives of registered nurses. *Jt Comm J Qual Patient Saf.* 2009;35:5–12.

Noting that health care is generally delivered by interdisciplinary teams (while discussions of disclosure of medical error tend to focus on physicians), this paper presents the findings of the first systematic study of nurses' attitudes toward and experiences with disclosure. Analyzing the results of focus groups (involving 96 RNs, representing multiple specialties in four institutions), the authors find that nurses routinely disclose minor nursing errors to their patients. However, nurses expect the physician to coordinate disclosure of serious and/or multidisciplinary errors and to involve nurses in the process. They note that often these expectations are not met. Because they are not informed of "what happened" and "what has been said," nurses feel that their ability to communicate honestly with patients is compromised. The study also reveals that nurse managers play a pivotal role in disclosure; nurses are more apt to disclose errors if the nurse manager takes a system approach to error and avoids assigning "blame." Nurses are generally unaware of existing institutional disclosure policies; nonetheless, nurses believe that policies that set expectations for professional collaboration regarding error would be helpful. Based on the findings, the authors make several recommendations, including (1) adoption of an institutional policy that fosters team disclosure, validates the role of the nurse, and protects those who raise concerns and (2) the development of a cadre of trained nurse managers with experience in disclosure. Fostering a team approach to error disclosure may help reduce the gap between the goal of disclosure and actual practice.

Waterman AD, Garbutt J, Hazel E, et al. The emotional impact of medical errors on practicing physicians in the United States and Canada. *Jt Comm J Qual Patient Saf.* 2007;33:467–476.

A survey of how physicians' experiences with medical error affect job satisfaction was completed by 1,767 American physicians and 1,414 Canadian physicians. Among the results reported was the fact that 92 percent of the physicians had been involved with an error or a near miss. Of the physicians surveyed, 89 percent reported having disclosed a serious error to a patient (although few had received training in how to conduct the conversation). Approximately half of the physicians reported that involvement in medical error increased their job-related stress. (Factors contributing to increased stress included the severity of the error, the perception of the likelihood of being sued, and feelings of lack of support.) There was widespread dissatisfaction with the support received from health care institutions after an error was made and interest in further training.

Wu AW, Folkman S, McPhee SJ, Lo B. Do house officers learn from their mistakes? *JAMA.* 1991;265:2089–2094.

Wu and colleagues surveyed internal medicine trainees (114 completed questionnaires) in large tertiary care facilities about the most serious mistake each had made in the past year, including questions about the trainees' sense of responsibility, emotional reaction, discussions with others about the error, institutional response, and subsequent changes in practice. Slightly more than half the trainees reported discussing the error with the attending; 88 percent reported talking with another physician; and 24 percent told the patient/family. Trainees generally reported changes in practice in response to the event. Among the factors associated with constructive changes were accepting responsibility and discussing the error; one factor associated with defensive changes was a "judgmental" response from the institution. The authors make recommendations for promoting constructive learning and also suggest that attending physicians could serve as role models for trainees in disclosure discussions with patient/families.

Disclosure of Medical Error and the Law

Cohen JR. Toward candor after medical error: the first apology law. *Harvard Health Policy Review.* Spring 2004;5:21–24.

Cohen notes that under traditional evidentiary law, statements by parties to a case can be admitted as evidence against them. However, starting in 1986, several states enacted statutes that excluded from evidence certain expressions of sympathy after adverse medical outcomes. Colorado's law went further and provided that statements or conduct by a health care provider or employee expressing fault (as well as sympathy or compassion) cannot be used against the provider in a malpractice action. While noting that there are pros and cons to all "apology" laws, Cohen focuses on the potential implications of the Colorado statute, such as (1) encouragement of full disclosure and apology, (2) possible decrease in the incidence of suits, and (3) improved patient safety.

McDonnell WM, Guenther E. Narrative review: do state laws make it easier to say "I'm sorry"? *Ann Intern Med.* 2008;149:811–816.

The authors note that while the benefits of disclosure of medical error are well recognized, many physicians still do not disclose errors to their patients. One barrier to physician disclosure of medical error is fear that statements of empathy or responsibility will be used against the provider in a malpractice action. To help educate physicians about efforts that have been taken to reduce this risk, the authors identify and analyze all laws in the United States and the District of Columbia (as of March 31, 2008) that prevent certain statements from being used against a provider at trial. They include information on what types of statements are protected under each law. In regard to those states without laws, the authors note that because apology laws are relatively new, the effects of such laws (such as reduced litigation or improved communication) are as yet unclear. Thus, the authors cannot make evidence-based recommendations as to new apology laws. Nonetheless, physicians in these states can work with legislators to craft laws that may meet their needs.

Taft L. Apology and medical mistake: opportunity or foil? *Annals of Health Law.* 2005;14:55–94.

Taft, an experienced patient-plaintiff attorney, is critical of those who urge "disclosure" but at the same time advise providers to avoid acknowledging and apologizing for medical error. Such advisers may use the word "apology," but they are referring to general expressions of empathy, which are designed in part to defend against liability. He contrasts such "pseudo apologies" with "authentic apologies," which are characterized by acknowledgment of the legitimacy of a norm that has been violated and fault in violating the norm; genuine remorse and regret; some attempt at restitution; an invitation for the injured party to forgive; and a willingness to accept the consequences of acknowledging fault. (He illustrates the difference between empathy and apology using existing disclosure policies.) Taft also criticizes "apology laws" in part because they encourage pseudo apologies. He suggests that such laws are based on a somewhat distorted view of malpractice litigation. In his experience, most cases involving potential liability are not accepted by plaintiffs' attorneys because the costs are high and the likelihood of victory small. If a case is accepted, a physician's failure to apologize may actually work against him or her at trial. Further, cases involving clear negligence should not go to trial but should be settled. He suggests that future laws should promote settlements of legitimate claims without litigation. (Despite his support of authentic apologies, Taft acknowledges that such apologies could be used in some circumstances against the provider and recognizes that offering such apologies constitutes an act of moral integrity and courage.)

Disclosure and Guidelines, Programs and Recommendations

Veterans Health Administration. VHA Directive 2008-002, Disclosure of Adverse Events to Patients. January 18, 2008. www1.va.gov/vhapublications/ViewPublication.asp?pub_ID=1637. Accessed April 10, 2010.

The VA was a leader in the development of disclosure policies. Its policy requires disclosure to patients or patients' representatives of adverse events even if the harm is not obvious or severe or may become evident only in the future. The policy divides disclosure into three types. "Clinical disclosure" is part of standard clinical care and is the responsibility of the attending physician and the clinical team. Clinical disclosure includes presenting the facts, expressing concern for the patient, and reassuring him or her that steps are being taken to prevent recurrence. "Institutional disclosure" occurs when the adverse event has resulted in death, serious harm, or potential liability and generally results in involvement of organization leaders and counsel. "Large scale disclosures" involve a large number of patients and require collaboration with the Department of Veterans Affairs Central Office. (Policy appendixes include further information, such as what events require disclosure, timing of disclosure, how disclosures should be made, and documentation.)

The Full Disclosure Working Group. *When Things Go Wrong: Responding to Adverse Events. A Consensus Statement of the Harvard Hospitals.* Boston: Massachusetts Coalition for the Prevention of Medical Errors; 2006.

This consensus statement of the Harvard teaching hospitals and the Risk Management Foundation contains clear and specific recommendations, supported by available data, expert opinion (including widely accepted ethical principles), and reasoning. The first section describes four essential steps in communicating with the patient/family (tell what happened, take responsibility, apologize, and explain what will be done to prevent future harm); suggestions regarding "who" should disclose, "when," and "how"; and recommendations for supporting the patient/family (including asking about their feelings and anxieties; providing names and addresses for follow-up questions; and addressing possible needs for financial support). The second section deals with the caregiver experience and recommends that institutions have a flexible program for providing support to clinicians (as well as offering training and education). The third section addresses management of the event, including elements of a hospital incident policy, analysis of the event, and documentation. In appendixes, the brochure offers model language for communicating with patients/family; a case study; and additional elements of caregiver support.

Joint Commission on Accreditation of Health Care Organizations. *Disclosing Medical Error: A Guide to an Effective Explanation and Apology.* Oakbrook Terrace, IL: Joint Commission Resources; 2007.

After a brief introduction to the incidence of medical error, this guide succinctly presents information and advice on reporting medical errors and on disclosing them to patients and families. The guide uses case studies to support its recommendations and to provide specific examples of ways to disclose error in a sensitive and compassionate manner. It posits that disclosure will reduce rather than increase costs arising from patient harm, but it also presents the counterarguments. The guide cites key references, including Web sites.

Shapiro E. Disclosing medical errors: best practices from the "leading edge." March 2008. www.ihi.org/IHI/Topics/PatientSafety/SafetyGeneral/Literature. Accessed January 22, 2009.

This paper details the leading efforts of medical institutions to foster open communication of medical error and to use what they learn from such communication to improve patient safety. Shapiro describes eight such institutions, including the process, the policy, training, outcomes, and lessons learned. Shapiro concludes that the experiences of organizations that pursue openness instead of acting in fear of lawsuits do not lead to increased suits but rather to greater satisfaction.

Woods MS. *Healing Words: The Power of Apology in Medicine.* Oak Park, IL: Doctors in Touch; 2004.

The author proposes that when complications occur in medical treatment, physicians should fully disclose what happened to the patient, apologize, and offer ongoing care and support. His position is based primarily on the physician's professional responsibility to treat the patient with respect and to obtain informed consent. He makes suggestions regarding an "authentic apology" (distinguished from a "compelled apology"). Woods also recognizes some of the barriers to acknowledging error, including the culture of medicine (with its emphasis on facts, data, and detachment) and malpractice concerns. While he believes that full and honest disclosure will reduce litigation, his argument is not dependent on such an outcome.

References

1. Institute of Medicine [U.S.]. Committee on Quality of Health Care in America. *To Err Is Human: Building a Safer Health System.* Washington, DC: National Academy Press; 2000.

2. Clinton HR, Obama B. Making patient safety the centerpiece of medical liability reform. *N Engl J Med.* 2006;354:2205–2208.

3. Hilfiker D. Facing our mistakes. *N Engl J Med.* 1984;310:118–122.

4. Bosk CL. *Forgive and Remember: Managing Medical Failure.* 2nd ed. Chicago: University of Chicago Press; 2003.

5. Wu AW. Medical error: the second victim. The doctor who makes the mistake needs help too. *BMJ.* 2000;320:726–727.

6. The Full Disclosure Working Group. *When Things Go Wrong: Responding to Adverse Events. A Consensus Statement of the Harvard Hospitals.* Boston: Massachusetts Coalition for the Prevention of Medical Errors; 2006.

7. Weingart SN. Beyond Babel: prospects for a universal patient safety taxonomy. *Int J Qual Health Care.* 2005;17:93–94.

8. Reason JT. *Human Error.* Cambridge, England: Cambridge University Press; 1990.

9. Quality Interagency Coordination Task Force. *Doing What Counts for Patient Safety: Federal Actions to Reduce Medical Errors and Their Impact.* February 2000. www.quic.gov/report/toc.htm. Accessed December 11, 2002.

10. Smith ML, Forster HP. Morally managing medical mistakes. *Camb Q Healthc Ethic.* 2000; 9:38–53.

11. Crigger NJ. Always having to say you're sorry: an ethical response to making mistakes in professional practice. *Nurs Ethics.* 2004;11:568–576.

12. Espin S, Levinson W, Regehr G, Baker GR, Lingard L. Error or "act of God"? a study of patients' and operating room team members' perceptions of error definition, reporting, and disclosure. *Surgery.* 2006;139:6–14.

13. Kuzel AJ, Woolf SH, Gilchrist VJ, et al. Patient reports of preventable problems and harms in primary health care. *Ann Fam Med.* 2004;2:333–340.

14. Burroughs TE, Waterman AD, Gallagher TH, et al. Patients' concerns about medical errors during hospitalization. *Jt Comm J Qual Saf.* 2007;33:5–14.

15. Gallagher TH, Waterman AD, Ebers AG, Fraser VJ, Levinson W. Patients' and physicians' attitudes regarding the disclosure of medical errors. *JAMA.* 2003;289:1001–1007.

16. Elder NC, Jacobson CJ, Zink T, Hasse L. How experiencing preventable medical problems changed patients' interactions with primary health care. *Ann Fam Med.* 2005;3:537–544.

17. Leape LL, Brennan TA, Laird N, et al. The nature of adverse events in hospitalized patients: results of the Harvard Medical Practice Study II. *N Engl J Med.* 1991;324:377–384.

18. Bates DW, Boyle DL, Vander Vliet MB, Schneider J, Leape L. Relationship between medication errors and adverse drug events. *J Gen Intern Med.* 1995;10:199–205.

19. Banja JD. Problematic medical errors and their implications for disclosure. *HEC Forum.* 2008;20:201–213.

20. Wu AW, Cavanaugh TA, McPhee SJ, Lo B, Micco GP. To tell the truth: ethical and practical issues in disclosing medical mistakes to patients. *J Gen Intern Med.* 1997;12:770–775.

21. Gallagher TH, Levinson W. Disclosing harmful medical errors to patients: a time for professional action. *Arch Intern Med.* 2005;165:1819–1824.

22. Wachter R, Shojania K. *Internal Bleeding: The Truth behind America's Terrible Epidemic of Medical Mistakes.* New York: Rugged Land; 2005.

23. Kenney C. *The Best Practice: How the New Quality Movement Is Transforming Medicine.* New York: PublicAffairs; 2008.

24. Brennan TA, Leape LL, Laird NM, et al. Incidence of adverse events and negligence in hospitalized patients: results of the Harvard Medical Practice Study I. *N Engl J Med.* 1991;324:370–376.

25. Thomas EJ, Studdert DM, Burstin HR, et al. Incidence and types of adverse events and negligent care in Utah and Colorado. *Med Care.* 2000;38: 261–271.

26. Stelfox HT, Palmisani S, Scurlock C, Orav EJ, Bates DW. The "To Err Is Human" report and the patient safety literature. *Qual Saf Health Care.* 2006; 15:174–178.

27. Institute of Medicine [U.S.]. Committee on Quality of Health Care in America. *Crossing the Quality Chasm: A New Health System for the 21st Century.* Washington, DC: National Academy Press; 2001.

28. Chedoe I, Molendijk HA, Dittrich ST, et al. Incidence and nature of medication errors in neonatal intensive care with strategies to improve safety: a review of the current literature. *Drug Saf.* 2007;30:503–513.

29. Gurwitz JH, Field TS, Harrold LR, et al. Incidence and preventability of adverse drug events among older persons in the ambulatory setting. *JAMA.* 2003;289:1107–1116.

30. Holdsworth MT, Fichtl RE, Behta M, et al. Incidence and impact of adverse drug events in pediatric inpatients. *Arch Pediatr Adolesc Med.* 2003;157: 60–65.

31. Phillips DP, Bredder CC. Morbidity and mortality from medical errors: an increasingly serious public health problem. *Annu Rev Public Health.* 200;223: 135–150.

32. Seifert SA, Jacobitz K. Pharmacy prescription dispensing errors reported to a regional poison control center. *J Toxicol Clin Toxicol.* 2002;40:919–923.

33. Boyle D, O'Connell D, Platt FW, Albert RK. Disclosing errors and adverse events in the intensive care unit. *Crit Care Med.* May 2006;34:1532–1537.

34. Gallagher TH. Medical errors in the outpatient setting: ethics in practice. *J Clin Ethics.* 2002;13:291–300.

35. Rothschild JM, Landrigan CP, Cronin JW, et al. The Critical Care Safety Study: the incidence and nature of adverse events and serious medical errors in intensive care. *Crit Care Med.* 2005;33:1694–1700.

36. Zhan C, Miller MR. Excess length of stay, charges, and mortality attributable to medical injuries during hospitalization. *JAMA.* 2003;290:1868–1874.

37. HealthGrades. *HealthGrades Quality Study: Patient Safety in American Hospitals.* July 2004. www.healthgrades.com/press-releases/. Accessed August 18, 2009.

38. Facing up to medical error. *BMJ.* March 18, 2000;320:A.

39. Spath P, ed. *Error Reduction in Health Care: A Systems Approach to Improving Patient Safety.* Chicago: AHA Press/Jossey-Bass Publications; 2000.

40. Leonard M, Frankel A, Simmonds T, Vega K, eds. *Achieving Safe and Reliable Healthcare.* Chicago: Health Administration Press; 2004.

41. Six Sigma. What Is Six Sigma? www.isixsigma.com/. Accessed August 18, 2009.

42. Connor M, Duncombe D, Barclay E, et al. Creating a fair and just culture: one institution's path toward organizational change. *Jt Comm J Qual Saf.* 2007;33:617–624.

43. Marx D. *Patient Safety and the "Just Culture": A Primer for Health Care Executives.* New York: Trustees of Columbia University; 2001. www.mers-tm .org/support/Marx_Primer.pdf. Accessed April 23, 2010.

44. AHRQ. Patient safety culture surveys. www.ahrq.gov/QUAL/patient safetyculture/. Accessed August 18, 2009.

45. *The National Medical Error Disclosure and Compensation Act.* S 1784, 109th Cong, 1st Sess (2005).

46. *The Patient Safety and Quality Improvement Act of 2005.* Overview, June 2008. Agency for Healthcare Research and Quality, Rockville, MD. www.ahrq.gov/qual/psoact.htm. Accessed April 10, 2010.

47. CMS. Physician Quality Reporting Initiative. www.cms.hhs.gov/pqri/. Accessed August 18, 2009.

48. National Academy for State Health Policy. www.nashp.org. Accessed April 20, 2010.

49. Kaiser Family Foundation. Spotlight: Personal experiences with medical errors. www.kff.org/spotlight/mederrors/4.cfm. Accessed August 18, 2009.

50. Blendon RJ, DesRoches CM, Brodie M, et al. Views of practicing physicians and the public on medical errors. *N Engl J Med.* 2002;347:1933–1940.

51. The Kaiser Family Foundation/Agency for Healthcare Research and Quality/Harvard School of Public Health. *National Survey on Consumers' Experiences with Patient Safety and Quality Information.* November 2004. www.kff.org/kaiserpolls/upload/National-Survey-on-Consumers-Experiences-With-Patient-Safety-and-Quality-Information-Survey-Summary-and-Chartpack.pdf. Accessed March 27, 2007.

52. HealthGrades. *Second Annual Patient Safety in American Hospitals Report.* May 2005. patientsafetyinamericanhospitalsreportfinal42905post.pdf from www.healthgrades.com. Accessed April 10, 2010.

53. AHRQ. *National Healthcare Quality Report*, 2008. www.ahrq.gov/qual/nhrq08/nhrq08.pdf. Accessed April 10, 2010.

54. HealthGrades. *The Eleventh Annual HealthGrades Hospital Quality in America Study.* October 2008. www.healthgrades.com/media/DMS/pdf/HealthGradesEleventhAnnualHospitalQualityStudy2008.pdf. Accessed April 10, 2010.

55. Altman DE, Clancy C, Blendon RJ. Improving patient safety—five years after the IOM report. *N Engl J Med.* 2004;351:2041–2043.

56. Wachter RM. The end of the beginning: patient safety five years after "To Err Is Human." *Health Aff* (Millwood). 2004;W4:534–545.

57. Berwick DM. Errors today and errors tomorrow. *N Engl J Med.* 2003;348:2570–2572.

58. Leape LL, Berwick DM. Five years after To Err Is Human: what have we learned? *JAMA.* 2005;293:2384–2390.

59. AHRQ. *2007 National Healthcare Quality & Disparities Reports.* www.ahrq.gov/qual/qrdr07.htm. Accessed August 18, 2009.

60. Ulmer C, Wolman D, Johns M. *Resident Duty Hours: Enhancing Sleep, Supervision, and Safety.* Washington, DC: National Academies of Science; 2009.

61. Buerhaus P. Is hospital patient care becoming safer? a conversation with Lucian Leape. *Health Aff* (Millwood). 2007;26:w687–w696.

62. Pronovost P, Needham D, Berenholtz S, et al. An intervention to decrease catheter-related bloodstream infections in the ICU. *N Engl J Med.* 2006; 355:2725–2732.

63. Cincinati Children's Hospital. Pursuing perfect care. www.cincinnati childrens.org/about/measures/perfect.htm. Accessed August 18, 2009.

64. Lee TH, Torchiana DF, Lock JE. Is zero the ideal death rate? *N Engl J Med.* 2007;357:111–113.

65. Leape L. Personal communication with Robert Truog, March 4, 2009.

66. Hobgood C, Peck CR, Gilbert B, Chappell K, Zou B. Medical errors—what and when: what do patients want to know? *Acad Emerg Med.* 2002;9: 1156–1161.

67. Hobgood C, Tamayo-Sarver JH, Elms A, Weiner B. Parental preferences for error disclosure, reporting, and legal action after medical error in the care of their children. *Pediatrics.* 2005;116:1276–1286.

68. Mazor KM, Simon SR, Gurwitz JH. Communicating with patients about medical errors: a review of the literature. *Arch Intern Med.* 2004;164: 1690–1697.

69. Witman AB, Park DM, Hardin SB. How do patients want physicians to handle mistakes? a survey of internal medicine patients in an academic setting. *Arch Intern Med.* 1996;156:2565–2569.

70. Mazor KM, Simon SR, Yood RA, et al. Health plan members' views about disclosure of medical errors. *Ann Intern Med.* 2004;140:409–418.

71. Mazor KM, Simon SR, Yood RA, et al. Health plan members' views on forgiving medical errors. *Am J Manag Care.* 2005;11:49–52.

72. Duclos CW, Eichler M, Taylor L, et al. Patient perspectives of patient-provider communication after adverse events. *Int J Qual Health Care.* 2005;17: 479–486.

73. American Society for Healthcare Risk Management of the American Hospital Association. Disclosure of unanticipated events: the next step in better communication with patients [first of three parts]. May 2003. www.ashrm.org/ashrm/resources/monograph.html. Accessed June 12, 2008.

74. Berlinger N. *After Harm: Medical Error and the Ethics of Forgiveness.* Baltimore, MD: Johns Hopkins University Press; 2005.

75. Lazare A. *On Apology.* Oxford, England: Oxford University Press; 2004.

76. Mazor KM, Reed GW, Yood RA, Fischer MA, Baril J, Gurwitz JH. Disclosure of medical errors: what factors influence how patients respond? *J Gen Intern Med.* 2006;21:704–710.

77. Robbennolt JK. Apologies and legal settlement: an empirical examination. *Michigan Law Review.* 2003;102:460–516.

78. Cleopas A, Villaveces A, Charvet A, Bovier PA, Kolly V, Perneger TV. Patient assessments of a hypothetical medical error: effects of health outcome, disclosure, and staff responsiveness. *Qual Saf Health Care.* April 2006;15:136–141.

79. Bismark M, Dauer E, Paterson R, Studdert D. Accountability sought by patients following adverse events from medical care: the New Zealand experience. *CMAJ.* 2006;175:889–894.

80. Hickson GB, Federspiel CF, Pichert JW, Miller CS, Gauld-Jaeger J, Bost P. Patient complaints and malpractice risk. *JAMA.* 2002;287:2951–2957.

81. Kachalia A, Shojania KG, Hofer TP, Piotrowski M, Saint S. Does full disclosure of medical errors affect malpractice liability? the jury is still out. *Jt Comm J Qual Saf.* 2003;29:503–511.

82. May ML, Stengel DB. Who sues their doctors? how patients handle medical grievances. *Law & Society Review.* 1990;24:105–120.

83. Vincent C, Young M, Phillips A. Why do people sue doctors? a study of patients and relatives taking legal action. *Lancet.* 1994;343:1609–1613.

84. Banja JD. *Medical Errors and Medical Narcissism.* Sudbury, MA: Jones and Bartlett Publishers; 2004.

85. Hebert PC, Levin AV, Robertson G. Bioethics for clinicians: 23. disclosure of medical error. *CMAJ.* 2001;164:509–513.

86. *When Things Go Wrong: Voices of Patients and Families* [DVD]. Cambridge, MA: CRICO/RMF; 2006.

87. Gibson R, Singh JP. *Wall of Silence: The Untold Story of the Medical Mistakes That Kill and Injure Millions of Americans.* Washington, DC: LifeLine Press; 2003.

88. Gawande A. *Complications: A Surgeon's Notes on an Imperfect Science.* New York: Metropolitan Books; 2002.

89. Levinson W, Dunn PM. A piece of my mind: coping with fallibility. *JAMA.* 1989;261:2252.

90. American Medical Association Council on Ethical and Judicial Affairs. *Code of Medical Ethics, Annotated Current Opinions.* 2004–2005 ed. Chicago, IL: American Medical Association.

91. American Nurses Association. Code of Ethics for Nurses. Section 3.4 "Standards and review mechanisms. www.nursingworld.org/mainmenuCategories/EthicsStandards. Accessed April 10, 2010.

92. Snyder L, Leffler C. Ethics manual: fifth edition. *Ann Intern Med.* 2005; 142:560–582.

93. Medical professionalism in the new millennium: a physician charter. *Ann Intern Med.* 2002;136:243–246.

94. American College of Surgeons. Code of Professional Conduct. www.facs.org/memberservices/codeofconduct.html. Accessed April 10, 2010.

95. Gallagher TH, Denham C, Leape L, Amori G, Levinson W. Disclosing unanticipated outcomes to patients: the art and the practice. *J Patient Safety.* 2007;3:158–165.

96. Gallagher TH, Studdert D, Levinson W. Disclosing harmful medical errors to patients. *N Engl J Med.* 2007;356:2713–2719.

97. Garbutt J, Waterman AD, Kapp JM, et al. Lost opportunities: how physicians communicate about medical errors. *Health Aff* (Millwood). 2008;27: 246–255.

98. Wu AW, Folkman S, McPhee SJ, Lo B. Do house officers learn from their mistakes? *JAMA.* 1991;265:2089–2094.

99. Gallagher TH, Garbutt JM, Waterman AD, et al. Choosing your words carefully: how physicians would disclose harmful medical errors to patients. *Arch Intern Med.* 2006;166:1585–1593.

100. Gallagher TH, Waterman AD, Garbutt JM, et al. US and Canadian physicians' attitudes and experiences regarding disclosing errors to patients. Arch Intern Med. 2006; 166:1605–1611.

101. Kaldjian LC, Forman-Hoffman VL, Jones EW, Wu BJ, Levi BH, Rosenthal GE. Do faculty and resident physicians discuss their medical errors? *J Med Ethics.* 2008;34:717–722.

102. Kaldjian LC, Jones EW, Wu BJ, Forman-Hoffman VL, Levi BH, Rosenthal GE. Disclosing medical errors to patients: attitudes and practices of physicians and trainees. *J Gen Intern Med.* 2007;22:988–996.

103. Chan DK, Gallagher TH, Reznick R, Levinson W. How surgeons disclose medical errors to patients: a study using standardized patients. *Surgery.* 2005;138: 851–858.

104. Fein SP, Hilborne LH, Spiritus EM, et al. The many faces of error disclosure: a common set of elements and a definition. *J Gen Intern Med.* 2007; 22:755–761.

105. Robinson AR, Hohmann KB, Rifkin JI, et al. Physician and public opinions on quality of health care and the problem of medical errors. *Arch Intern Med.* 2002;162:2186–2190.

106. Gilbert S. *Wrongful Death: A Memoir.* New York: W. W. Norton; 1997.

107. Katz J. Why doctors don't disclose uncertainty. *Hastings Cent Rep.* February 1984;14:35–44.

108. Baylis F. Errors in medicine: nurturing truthfulness. *J Clin Ethics.* 1997;8:336–340.

109. Mizrahi T. Managing medical mistakes: ideology, insularity and accountability among internists-in-training. *Soc Sci Med.* 1984;19:135–146.

110. White AA, Gallagher TH, Krauss MJ, et al. The attitudes and experiences of trainees regarding disclosing medical errors to patients. *Acad Med.* 2008;83:250–256.

111. Waterman AD, Garbutt J, Hazel E, et al. The emotional impact of medical errors on practicing physicians in the United States and Canada. *Jt Comm J Qual Saf.* 2007;33:467–476.

112. Orlander JD, Barber TW, Fincke BG. The morbidity and mortality conference: the delicate nature of learning from error. *Acad Med.* 2002;77:1001–1006.

113. Pierluissi E, Fischer MA, Campbell AR, Landefeld CS. Discussion of medical errors in morbidity and mortality conferences. *JAMA.* 2003;290: 2838–2842.

114. White A, Waterman A, McCotter P, Boyle D, Gallagher T. Supporting healthcare workers after medical errors: considerations for health care leaders. *J Clinical Outcomes Management.* 2008;15:240–247.

115. Christensen JF, Levinson W, Dunn PM. The heart of darkness: the impact of perceived mistakes on physicians. *J Gen Intern Med.* 1992;7: 424–431.

116. Taft L. On bended knee (with fingers crossed). *Depaul Law Review.* 2005;55:601–616.

117. Brennan TA, Sox CM, Burstin HR. Relation between negligent adverse events and the outcomes of medical-malpractice litigation. *N Engl J Med.* 1996; 335:1963–1967.

118. Brennan TA, Mello MM. Patient safety and medical malpractice: a case study. *Ann Intern Med.* 2003;139:267–273.

119. Dauer E. A therapeutic jurisprudence perspective on legal responses to medical error. *J Legal Med.* 2003;24:37–50.

120. Sharpe V. *Accountability: Patient Safety and Policy Reform.* Washington, DC: Georgetown University Press; 2004.

121. Mello MM, Studdert DM, Brennan TA. The new medical malpractice crisis. *N Engl J Med.* 2003;348:2281–2284.

122. Studdert DM, Mello MM, Brennan TA. Medical malpractice. *N Engl J Med.* 2004;350:283–292.

123. Studdert DM, Mello MM, Gawande AA, et al. Claims, errors, and compensation payments in medical malpractice litigation. *N Engl J Med.* 2006; 354:2024–2033.

124. Banja J. *Does Medical Error Disclosure Violate the Medical Malpractice Cooperation Clause? Advances in Patient Safety.* Vol 3. Washington, DC: AHRQ; 2005.

125. Cohen JR. Apology and organizations: exploring an example from medical practice. *Fordham Urban Law Journal.* 2000;27:1447–1482.

126. Levinson W, Roter DL, Mullooly JP, Dull VT, Frankel RM. Physician-patient communication: the relationship with malpractice claims among primary care physicians and surgeons. *JAMA.* 1997;277:553–559.

127. Wojcieszak D, Banja J, Houk C. The Sorry Works! Coalition: making the case for full disclosure. *Jt Comm J Qual Saf.* 2006;32:344–350.

128. Wojcieszak D, Saxton JW, Finkelstein MM. Ethics training needs to emphasize disclosure and apology. *HEC Forum.* 2008;20:291–305.

129. Popp PL. How will disclosure affect future litigation? *J Healthc Risk Manag.* Winter 2003;23:5–9.

130. Boothman R, Blackwell A, Campbell D, Commiskey E, Anderson S. A better approach to medical malpractice claims? the University of Michigan experience. *J Health Life Sciences Law.* 2009;2:125–159.

131. Kraman SS, Cranfill L, Hamm G, Woodard T. John M. Eisenberg Patient Safety Awards. Advocacy: the Lexington Veterans Affairs Medical Center. *Jt Comm J Qual Improv.* 2002;28:646–650.

132. Kraman SS, Hamm G. Risk management: extreme honesty may be the best policy. *Ann Intern Med.* 1999;131:963–967.

133. McDonald T, Smith K, Chamberlin W, Centomani NM. Full disclosure is more than saying "I'm sorry." *Focus on Patient Safety.* 2009;11:1–3.

134. Testimony of Richard C. Boothman, Chief Risk Officer, University of Michigan Health System, before the Senate Committee on Health, Education and Labor and Pensions, June 22, 2006.

135. Studdert DM, Mello MM, Gawande AA, Brennan TA, Wang YC. Disclosure of medical injury to patients: an improbable risk management strategy. *Health Aff* (Millwood). 2007;26:215–226.

136. McDonnell WM, Guenther E. Narrative review: do state laws make it easier to say "I'm sorry?" *Ann Intern Med.* 2008;149:811–816.

137. Wei M. Doctors, apologies, and the law: an analysis and critique of apology laws. *J Health Law.* Fall 2006;39. www.ssrn.com/abstract=955668. Accessed March 27, 2007.

138. Shapiro E. Disclosing medical errors: best practices from the "leading edge." March 2008. www.ihi.org/IHI/Topics/PatientSafety/SafetyGeneral/Literature. Accessed January 22, 2009.

139. Gallagher TH. A 62-year-old woman with skin cancer who experienced wrong-site surgery: review of medical error. *JAMA*. 2009;302:669–677.

140. Cantor MD, Barach P, Derse A, Maklan CW, Wlody GS, Fox E. Disclosing adverse events to patients. *Jt Comm J Qual Saf*. January 2005;31:5–12.

141. Veterans Health Administration. VHA Directive 2008-002, Disclosure of Adverse Events to Patients. January 18, 2008. www1.va.gov/vhapublications/ViewPublication.asp?pub_ID=1637. Accessed April 10, 2010.

142. Shapiro J. Personal communication with Robert Truog, July 20, 2009.

143. Gallagher TH, Quinn R. What to do with the unanticipated outcome: does apologizing make a difference? how does early resolution impact settlement outcome? Medical liability and health care law seminar. Phoenix: Defense Research Institute; 2006.

144. Lamb RM, Studdert DM, Bohmer RM, Berwick DM, Brennan TA. Hospital disclosure practices: results of a national survey. *Health Aff* (Millwood). 2003;22:73–83.

145. Gallagher T, Brundage G, Bommarito KM, et al. Risk managers' attitudes and experiences regarding patient safety and error disclosure: a national survey. *J Healthc Risk Manag*. 2006;26:11–16.

146. Weick K. The aesthetic of imperfection in orchestras and organizations. In: Kamoche K, ed. *Organizational Improvisation*. New York: Routledge; 2002: 166–184.

147. Edmondson A. Psychological safety and learning behavior in working teams. *Administrative Science Quarterly*. 1999;44:350–383.

148. Branch WT, Jr. Use of critical incident reports in medical education: a perspective. *J Gen Intern Med*. November 2005;20:1063–1067.

149. Meyer EC, Sellers DE, Browning DM, McGuffie K, Solomon MZ, Truog RD. Difficult conversations: improving communication skills and relational abilities in health care. *Pediatr Crit Care Med*. May 2009;10:352–359.

150. Browning DM, Meyer EC, Truog RD, Solomon MZ. Difficult conversations in health care: cultivating relational learning to address the hidden curriculum. *Acad Med*. September 2007;82:905–913.

151. Cannon M, Edmondson A. Failing to learn and learning to fail (intelligently): how great organizations put failure to work to innovate and improve. Long Range Planning. 2005;38:299–319.

152. Carroll JS, Edmondson AC. Leading organisational learning in health care. *Qual Saf Health Care*. 2002;11:51–56.

153. deBurca S. The learning health care organization. *Int J Qual Health Care.* 2000; 12:457–458.

154. Berwick D. *Escape Fire: Lessons for the Future of Health Care.* New York: Commonwealth Fund; 2002.

155. Joint Commission on Accreditation of Healthcare Organizations. *Health Care at the Crossroads: Strategies for Improving the Medical Liability System and Preventing Patient Injury.* 2005. www.jointcommission.org. Accessed April 10, 2010.

156. Kemp EC, Floyd MR, McCord-Duncan E, Lang F. Patients prefer the method of "tell back-collaborative inquiry" to assess understanding of medical information. *J Am Board Fam Med.* 2008;21:24–30.

157. The Sorry Works! Coalition: About Us. www.sorryworks.net/about.phtml. Accessed April 10, 2010.

158. Lindsey T. "Sorry" seen as magic word to avoid suits. Associated Press. November 11, 2004.

159. Sack K. Doctors say "I'm sorry" before "See you in court." *New York Times.* May 18, 2008; National Desk.

160. Zimmerman R. Medical contrition: doctors' new tool to fight lawsuits; saying "I'm sorry." *Wall Street Journal.* May 18, 2004:A:1.

161. Lazare A. Apology in medical practice: an emerging clinical skill. *JAMA.* 2006;296:1401–1404.

162. Quill T, Arnold R, Platt FM. "I wish things were different": Expressing wishes in response to loss, futility, and unrealistic hopes. *Ann Intern Med.* 2001; 135:551–555.

163. Boland R, Tenkasi R. Perspective making and perspective taking in communities of knowing. *Organizational Science.* 1995;6:350–372.

164. Hall D, David R. Engaging multiple perspectives: a value-based decision-making model. *Decision Support Systems.* 2007;43:1588–1604.

165. Sessa V. Using perspective taking to manage conflict and affect in teams. *J Applied Behavioral Sciences.* 1996;32:101–115.

166. National Quality Forum. *Safe Practices for Better Healthcare—2009 Update: A Consensus Report.* Washington, DC: National Quality Forum; 2009.

167. Dintzis SM, Gallagher TH. Disclosing harmful pathology errors to patients. *Am J Clin Pathol.* 2009;131:463–465.

168. Holmqvist M. A dynamic model of intra- and interorganizational learning. *Organizational Studies.* 2003;24:95–123.

169. Weick K. Creativity and the aesthetics of imperfection. In: Ford C, Gioia D, eds. *Creative Action in Organizations.* Thousand Oaks, CA: Sage; 1995: 187–192.

170. Davidoff F. Shame: the elephant in the room. *BMJ*. 2002;324:623–624.

171. Inui T. *A Flag in the Wind: Educating for Professionalism in Medicine*. Washington, DC: Association of American Medical Colleges; 2003.

172. Loren DJ, Klein EJ, Garbutt J, et al. Medical error disclosure among pediatricians: choosing carefully what we might say to parents. *Arch Pediatr Adolesc Med*. 2008;162:922–927.

173. Shannon SE, Foglia MB, Hardy M, Gallagher TH. Disclosing errors to patients: perspectives of registered nurses. *Jt Comm J Qual Saf*. 2009;35:5–12.

Index

Page numbers in *italics* refer to figures and tables.

ability of organization to intervene, developing, *123*, 126–29
accountability: apology and, 71–72; ascribing for bad outcomes, 13–14; avoidance of, 32; communication about, 119–20; as core relational value, 67; definition of, *67*; following up and, 81; organizational, establishing, *123*, 125–26
Accreditation Council on Graduate Medical Education, 29
action, turning ability into, *123*, 129–30
actors in enactments, role of, 92, 93–94, 102
adverse events: communication about, 14; definitions of, 12–13, *13*; goal of reduction to zero, 29–30; measurement of, 16; moral and emotional salience of, 62–63; as part of health care, xiv; positive outcomes after, 99–100
aesthetics of imperfection, 118, 137
Agency for Healthcare Research and Quality (AHRQ): adverse event definition of, 12; first national report on, 25; hospital survey on patient safety culture, 27, *28*; IOM report and, 22; medical error definition of, 10–11; patient safety indicators, 26
agendas, setting, 84
AHRQ. *See* Agency for Healthcare Research and Quality
American Association for the Advancement of Science, 17
American College of Physicians, 36
American College of Surgeons, 36
American Medical Association: Code of Ethics, 36, 112; conference on patient safety and, 17
American Nurses Association, 36
American Society for Healthcare Risk Management (ASHRM): adverse event definition of, 12; on disclosure, 15; IOM report and, 24
apology: accountability and, 71–72; conveying, 86–87; types of, 70–72
apology laws, 50–51
ASHRM. *See* American Society for Healthcare Risk Management
ask-tell-ask method, 70, 77, 84–85
attention to medical needs of patients, ensuring, 75
attitude surveys, 123–24
autonomy, principle of, 34
aviation industry, response to errors within, 20–21
awareness of importance of disclosure, promotion of, 122–25, *123*

bad apple mentality, xiii, 17–18
Banja, John, 13, 41
Bataldan, Paul, 16
Berlinger, Nancy, 35
Berwick, Don, 16, 17, 66

blame: accepting, 99; act of assigning, 97–98, 126
Boothman, Richard, 46, 47
Brigham and Women's Hospital, *53*, 54–55

caring: apology as expression of, 70–71; conveying, 86–87; expressing, 82
casuistry, 103–4
Catholic Health Initiatives, 54
Chan, D. K., 39
change, importance of, vii–viii, 73
Children's Hospital Boston, 58
clinical disclosures, 52
clinicians: apologies from organizations to, 120; ask-tell-ask method and, 77; as coaches, 60; meeting needs of, 78–79, 90; primary conversations and, 61–62, 79; self-efficacy of, 101–2; support for, 127, 133–34; tendency to blame and, 97–98. *See also* physicians
Clinton, Hillary, xiv, 22, 47, *49*
coaching model of disclosure, 58–63
communication with patients: about adverse events, 14; acquisition of "skills" for, xvii–xviii; approaches to demonstrated in workshops, 96–101; challenges and complexity of, 57–58; as collaborative, 69–70, 84–85, 134–35; as in developmental infancy, 104–5; discrepancy between what is known and what is practiced in, viii; documentation of, 90–91; education and training for, 42, 136; elements of, 74–75; facts, stating, 80, 85–86, 96–97; following up after initial conversations, 81, 89, 127; illustration of breakdown in, 1–3; lawsuits and, xiv; needs and desires for, 31–33; timing of and settings for, 81, 106
compassion: conveying, 82, 83, 87; definition of, 68
compensation: acknowledging issues of, 88–89; offers of, 55, 134–35
conflict between ethical principles, 35, 72–73
"connect the dots" disclosures, 39
consequentialism, principle of, 34
Consumers Advancing Patient Safety, vii
context, effects of on disclosure conversations, 101
continuity: as core relational value, 67; definition of, *67*; following up and, 81; primary caregivers and, 80
conversations. *See* communication with patients
COPIC Insurance Company, *53*, 55, *56*, 134
Crigger, Nancy, 11
culture: of blame, 98; of silence, xiii, 18, 40–42
culture of health care institutions: as dysfunctional, viii; importance of change in, 56, 129–30, 137. *See also* culture, of silence
curriculum for disclosure coaches: core relational values and, 66–67; design of, 64–65; overview of, 62–63

"dashboards," 131
debriefing conversations, 90
"deferring" disclosures, 40
delays in diagnosis, 106
disclosure malfunction, viii
disclosure of error: barriers to, 121–22, *130*; benefits of, 37–38; categories of, 52; coaching model of, 58–63; effect of on clinicians, 43–44; effect of on malpractice litigation, 44–50; ethical norms regarding, 33–36; as exception rather than norm, 38–43; institutional support for, 59–62; integration of into institutional safety and quality programs, 131–33; levels of, xvi; programs and policies regarding, 51–56; safe practice guideline on, 59, *59*; terminology of, 14–15; threshold for, 78. *See also* guidelines for disclosure; nondisclosure
documentation in medical records: of conversations, 90–91; of reasons for nondisclosure, 110, 111
dosing errors, 107–8, 110–11

early compensation practices, 55
education and training: for communication with patients, 42, 136; medical,

culture of, 41–42. *See also* enactments; vignettes for workshops
empathy: conveying, 83, 87; taught as skill, 68–69
enactments: approaches to communication demonstrated in, 96–101; description of, 92–94; lessons learned from, 101–2; paradigmatic case for, 94–96, *95*; role of actors in, 92, 93–94. *See also* vignettes for workshops
equipment or devices, sequestering, 76
error, definitions of, 10, 12, 14. *See also* medical error
Error Reduction in Health Care, 20
ethical issues: characteristics of medical error, 11; competing ethics, 72–73; enactments in workshops and, 102; norms regarding disclosure of error, 33–36; professional standards and, 36
ethics consultation, 61, 128–29
evidentiary rules, changes in, 50–51

facts, stating, 80, 85–86, 96–97
families: including in initial conversations, 79–80; needs of, as primary, 72–73, 128–29; needs of, regarding communication, 31–33
federal government response to IOM report, 21–22
Fein, S. P., 39–40
following up after initial conversations, 81, 89, 127
Forster, H. P., 11
frequency of errors, 19

Gallagher, T. H., 38, 40, 58, 74, 112
Garbutt, J. M., 112
gathering information, 77
Geisinger Health System, *53*, 54
Gilbert, Sandra, 40
"Golden Rule," applying, 83, 113
guidelines for disclosure: first priorities, 75–76; overview of, 74–75, 139–40; preparation for conversation, 77–82

Harvard Medical Practice Study, 16
Harvard Medical School consensus document, 8, 57
Harvard Medical School–CRICO/RMF, *53*, 58
HealthGrades, 25
"hidden curriculum" in health care, 121
"High Reliability Organization," 20
Hilfiker, David, 3–4
honesty about clinical decisions, 116
huddles: postconversation, 90; preconversation, 77, 93
Human Error (Reason), 10, 19

informed consent, doctrine of, 34
Institute for Healthcare Improvement (IHI), 19, 23
Institute of Medicine (IOM): *Crossing the Quality Chasm*, 18–19; definitions of, 12–13; Quality of Health Care in America project, 17–19, *18*; reports of, 18–19. See also *To Err Is Human*
institutional disclosures, 52. *See also* organizational disclosure strategies
institutional support for disclosure, 59–62
interprofessional approach to disclosure, 127–28
investigations, performing and communicating about, 87–88
IOM. *See* Institute of Medicine

Joint Commission on Accreditation of Healthcare Organizations (JCAHO), 17, 23
Josie King Foundation, vii
justice, principle of, 34
"just-in-time" access to expertise, 58–59, 75

Kaiser Family Foundation, 19, 25
Kaiser Permanente, 52, *53*, 54
Kaldjian, L. C., 39
kindness, as core relational value, 67, *67*, 68
knowledge, theoretical vs. practical, 64

latent errors, 20
lawsuits: common precipitants of, xiv; delays in diagnosis and, 106; effect of disclosure on, 44–50; physician fear of, 40

Lazare, Aaron, 35
leadership and organizational learning, 118–19, 124–25
Leape, Lucian: on adverse events, 12; on calls for perfection, 30; on complex causes of error, 20; on disclosure and apology, 31, 57–58; IOM project and, 17; on residency programs, 29; on "second victims" of error, 43; *When Things Go Wrong* and, 57
Leapfrog Group for Patient Safety, 23–24, 27
learning from errors, 100–101. *See also* organizational learning
Lee, Thomas, 29
Lehman, Betsy, 16–17

malpractice insurers, collaboration between, 134–35
malpractice litigation, effect of disclosure on, 44–50
malpractice reform, xiv
Marx, David, 21
Mazor, K. M., 38
medical education and training, culture of, 41–42
medical error: definitions of, 10–15, *13*; Hilfiker on, 3–4; illustrations of, 1–2, 4–7, 8–9; as leading cause of death, xiii; new paradigm for thinking about, 17–18; as part of health care, xiv
Medically Induced Trauma Support Services (MITSS), vii, 24, 44, 89, 90
"Medical Professionalism in the New Millennium: A Physician Charter," 36
medical records, documentation in: about conversations, 90–91; about reasons for nondisclosure, 110, 111
Medicare program: financial incentives for error reduction in, 22; as source of data, 19
"misleading" disclosures, 39–40
MITSS (Medically Induced Trauma Support Services), vii, 24, 44, 89, 90
mixed messages, 121–22
Morbidity and Mortality conferences, 42–43, 99, 124
Mothers Against Medical Errors, vii

narrative ethics, 34–35
National Association of Children's Hospitals and Related Institutions (NACHRI), 27
National Guidelines Clearinghouse, 22
National Practitioner Data Bank, 135
National Quality Forum: coaching model of, 62; guidelines for conversations with patients, 74; IOM report and, 23; never events and, 27; safe practice guideline on disclosure, 59, *59*, 126
National Quality Measures Clearinghouse, 22
near misses: definition of, 13, *13*; disclosure of, 78
needs assessments, 123–24
negligence cases, 44–45
never events, 27
New England Journal of Medicine, xiv, 3, 4, 47, 49
nondisclosure: documentation of, 110, 111; erring on side of, 116–17; justifications for, 35–36; practice of, 38–43; threshold for, 86
notification of key individuals, ensuring, 75–76

Obama, Barack, xiv, 22, 47, 49
organizational disclosure strategies: creating accountability, 125–26; developing ability, 126–29; 4-A framework for, 122, *123*; promoting awareness, 122–25; turning ability into action, 129–30
organizational learning: aesthetics of imperfection and, 118; core relational values and, 122; definition of, 118; as focus of conversations, 100–101; individuals and systems, 119–20; leadership and, 118–19, 124–25; mixed messages and, 121–22
organizational support for disclosure, 59–62
outcome measures related to disclosure, 126

paradigmatic cases, 92, 94–96, *95*, 103
"partial" disclosures, 39

pathologists, role of, 112
patient advocacy groups, vii, 24
Patient Quality Reporting System, 22
patients: attitudes of about error disclosure, *33*; definition of medical error of, 11–12; needs of, as primary, 72–73, 81–82, 128–29; root cause analysis procedures and, 132; support for, 127. *See also* communication with patients; patient safety movement
Patient Safety and Quality Improvement Act, 22
patient safety movement: access to information and, 18; cultural change and, 37; driving concept behind, vii, xiii; residency practice and, 27, 29; response to *To Err Is Human* and, 18–25; sentinel report in, 17–18; standards and, 26–27; themes of, 19
peer-protected review mechanisms, 6, 42
perfection, expectations of, 3–4, 21, 29–30, 41
Persons United Limiting Substandards and Errors in Health Care, vii
perspectives, multiple, seeing and understanding, 72–73
physicians: attitudes of about error disclosure, *33*; curriculum for, 57–58; education and training of, 41–42; effect of medical errors on, 3–4, 5, 6, 7–8; fiduciary nature of relationships with patients, 34; peer review mechanisms for, 6, 42; as "second victims," 7, 43. *See also* communication with patients
planning for disclosure meetings, 76, 77–82, 93
plans of care, explaining, 87
positive outcomes after adverse events, 99–100
postconversation huddles, 90
preconversation huddles, 77, 93
private medical staffs and disclosure challenges, 126
process measures related to disclosure, 125
professional ethical standards, 36
ProMutual, 134
Pronovost, Peter, 29

Quality Interagency Coordination (QuIC) Task Force: adverse event definition of, 12; IOM report and, 21; medical error definition of, 11; near miss definition of, 13

radiologists, role of, 112
Rand Corporation, 19
rapid response teams, 61
Rattner, David, 7
Reason, James, 10, 19
reasoning from abstract general principles to specific cases, 103–4
relationships: core relational values in, 66–67, *67*, 83; fiduciary nature of physician-patient, 34; repair of, 44, 87, 89, 133–34; rupture in, xiv, 9, 102
research, filling gap in, 136–37
residency practice, 27, 29
respect: as core relational value, *67*; definition of, *67*; "Golden Rule" and, 83, 113; principle of, 34
responses to disclosure, 89–90, 129
risk managers, 60, 79
role modeling by disclosure coaches, 62–63
role playing, 80

safety programs, linking disclosure quality and, 131–33, 137
Salzberg, Sharon, 68
self-efficacy of clinicians, 101–2
sentinel cases, sharing, 124
Shapiro, Eve, 51–52, *53*
Shapiro, Jo, 54
Shtasel, Derri, 110
Six Sigma program, 21
sleep deprivation and residency programs, 29
Smith, M. L., 11
social workers, 79–80
"SorryWorks!", 24
Stanford University, *53*, 134
state government response to IOM report, 22–23
structure measures related to disclosure, 125–26
Studdert, D. M., 50
support services, offer of to patients and families, 89

support system for disclosure: for clinicians, 133–34; elements of, 126–29; institutional, 59–62
"swiss cheese" model of errors, 20
systems approaches to error reduction, 20–21. *See also* organizational disclosure strategies

team approach to disclosure, 127–28
terminology of book, 10–15
therapeutic exceptions, 86
timing of and settings for conversations, 81, 106
To Err Is Human (Institute of Medicine): definitions in, 12–13; description of, 17–18; progress five years after, 25–30; recommendations of, *18*; response to, 18–25
tort system, 44–45
TRACK. *See* values, core relational
transparency: capacity for, 120; as core relational value, 66–67; definition of, 67; honesty about clinical decisions and, 116; terminology for, 132
trust: breaches of, 102; rebuilding, 133–34

unintended consequences, risk of, 29
University of Illinois Medical Center, *53*, 134
University of Michigan, 46–47, 48, 49, *53*, 134

values, core relational: conflict among, 104; kindness, 68; living up to, 133–34; organizational learning and, 122; overview of, 66–67, *67*; rebuilding relationships and, 83, 102
Veterans Administration: Medical Center, Lexington, Kentucky, 46, 52, *53*; patient safety conference and, 17
vignettes for workshops: disconnected CVL, 108–10; DKA protocol, 115–17; dosing errors, 107–8, 110–11; error made at referring hospital, 111–12; overview of, 103–5; potassium level, 113–14; problem with new device, 112–13; PSA level, 105–7; wound infection, 114–15

Waterman, A. D., 112
Weick, Karl, 118
West Virginia Mutual, 134
When Things Go Wrong (film), 40–41
When Things Go Wrong: Responding to Adverse Events (Harvard consensus document), 8, 57
withholding of information about errors, 6
Wojciezak, Doug, 24
workshops: approaches to communication demonstrated in, 96–101; description of, 92–94; lessons learned from, 101–2; paradigmatic case for, 94–96, *95*; senior leaders and, 125. *See also* vignettes for workshops
Wu, Albert, 14, 38

zero tolerance level for error, 21, 29–30
Zion, Libby, 27

About the Authors

ROBERT D. TRUOG, M.D., is a professor of medical ethics, anaesthesiology, and pediatrics at Harvard Medical School. He has practiced pediatric intensive care medicine at Children's Hospital Boston for more than 20 years, and he has published more than 200 articles in bioethics and related disciplines. As director of Clinical Ethics at Harvard Medical School, he has a leadership role in teaching ethics across the undergraduate curriculum. As executive director of the Institute for Professionalism and Ethical Practice, he creates and teaches highly interactive seminars to enhance the relational and communication skills of clinicians across a variety of topics, including breaking bad news, discussing organ donation with families, and disclosure of adverse events and medical error. As chair of Harvard's Embryonic Stem Cell Research Oversight Committee (ESCRO), he is engaged in the interesting and difficult challenges of defining the ethical parameters of stem cell research.

DAVID M. BROWNING is a senior scholar at the Institute for Professionalism and Ethical Practice at Children's Hospital Boston and a lecturer at Harvard Medical School. His work as a medical educator focuses on promoting collaborative learning to bring about enhanced professionalism, improved clinical practice, and organizational change. At Children's, he is a member of the Ethics Advisory Committee and a recent recipient of the Medical Educator Award for Innovative Scholarship in Medical Education. Previously, Mr. Browning was a senior research scientist at Education Development Center, Inc., where he directed the Initiative for Pediatric Palliative Care, an interdisciplinary educational program for clinicians serving children with life-threatening conditions and their families. Mr. Browning is a recipient of the Social Work Leadership Development Award from the Open Society Institute. His recent publications have focused on improving everyday ethics in healthcare communication and front-line practice.

JUDITH A. JOHNSON received her undergraduate degree from Brown University and her law degree from Boston College Law School. She practiced health law in Boston for over 20 years. She was in private practice at the firms of Ropes & Gray and Choate, Hall & Stewart and served as vice president for Legal Services at New England Medical Center Hospitals. She received a Certificate in Health Care Ethics from the University of Washington School of Medicine and completed an ethics fellowship in the Division of Medical Ethics at Harvard Medical School. She is an Associate Clinical Ethicist at Children's Hospital Boston and serves on the Ethics Advisory Committee. She is a member of the Harvard Ethics Leadership Group and engages in teaching, research, and writing on legal and ethical issues.

THOMAS H. GALLAGHER, M.D., is a general internist and an associate professor in the Department of Medicine and the Department of Bioethics and Humanities at the University of Washington School of Medicine. He received his medical training from Harvard Medical School, did his medicine residency at Washington University in St. Louis, and completed a fellowship at the University of California San Francisco. Dr. Gallagher's research addresses the interfaces among health care quality, communication, and transparency, and he has published over 40 articles and book chapters on patient safety and error disclosure; his articles have appeared in leading journals including *JAMA, New England Journal of Medicine,* and *Health Affairs*. Dr. Gallagher is the principal investigator on two grants from the Agency for Healthcare Research and Quality, including a large AHRQ demonstration project entitled "Communication to Prevent and Respond to Medical Injuries: Washington State Collaborative." He also is a principal investigator on grants from the National Cancer Institute, the Robert Wood Johnson Foundation, and the Greenwall Foundation. He has conducted over 200 disclosure training sessions in the U.S. and abroad.